A PLUME BOOK

THE BRAIN POWER COOKBOOK

DR. FRANK LAWLIS is a renowned psychologist, researcher, and counselor with more than thirty-five years' experience working with families. He is the cofounder of the Lawlis and Peavey Centers for Psychoneurological Change and was named a fellow by the American Psychological Association. The chief content advisor for *The Dr. Phil Show*, Dr. Lawlis is also the author of *The Stress Answer, The ADD Answer, The IQ Answer,* and *Mending the Broken Bond.* He lives in Sanger, Texas.

DR. MAGGIE GREENWOOD-ROBINSON is a popular health and medical writer, and the author of *The Biggest Loser*, a *New York Times* bestseller that is the official diet/fitness book for NBC's hit reality show by the same name. She is author or coauthor of more than forty books on nutrition, exercise, weight loss, brain fitness, and health issues such as cancer, including *Good Foods vs Bad Foods and 20/20 Thinking.* Maggie is a member of the Dr. Phil show Advisory Board and serves on the Advisory Board of *Physical Magazine.*

The
BRAIN POWER
COOKBOOK

More Than 200 Recipes to
Energize Your Thinking,
Boost Your Mood, and
Sharpen Your Memory

Dr. FRANK LAWLIS
and
Dr. MAGGIE GREENWOOD-ROBINSON

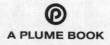

A PLUME BOOK

PLUME
Published by the Penguin Group
Penguin Group (USA) Inc., 375 Hudson Street, New York, New York 10014, U.S.A. • Penguin
Group (Canada), 90 Eglinton Avenue East, Suite 700, Toronto, Ontario, Canada M4P 2Y3 (a
division of Pearson Penguin Canada Inc.) • Penguin Books Ltd., 80 Strand, London WC2R
0RL, England • Penguin Ireland, 25 St. Stephen's Green, Dublin 2, Ireland (a division of
Penguin Books Ltd.) • Penguin Group (Australia), 250 Camberwell Road, Camberwell,
Victoria 3124, Australia (a division of Pearson Australia Group Pty. Ltd.) • Penguin Books
India Pvt. Ltd., 11 Community Centre, Panchsheel Park, New Delhi – 110 017, India • Penguin
Group (NZ), 67 Apollo Drive, Rosedale, North Shore 0632, New Zealand (a division of Pearson
New Zealand Ltd) • Penguin Books (South Africa) (Pty.) Ltd., 24 Sturdee Avenue, Rosebank,
Johannesburg 2196, South Africa

Penguin Books Ltd., Registered Offices: 80 Strand, London WC2R 0RL, England

First published by Plume, a member of Penguin Group (USA) Inc.

First Printing, January 2009
10   9   8   7   6   5   4   3   2   1

 REGISTERED TRADEMARK—MARCA REGISTRADA

LIBRARY OF CONGRESS CATALOGING-IN-PUBLICATION DATA
Lawlis, G. Frank
   The brain power cookbook : more than 200 recipes to energize your thinking, boost your mood,
and sharpen your memory / Frank Lawlis and Maggie Greenwood-Robinson.
      p. cm.
   Includes index.
   ISBN 978-0-452-29013-6 (trade pbk.)
   1. Intellect—Nutritional aspects.   2. Cookery.   3. Mental health—Nutritional aspects.
I. Greenwood-Robinson, Maggie.   II Title.
RC455.4.N8L388   2009
641.5'63—dc22   2008025127

Printed in the United States of America
Set in Goudy Old Style
Designed by Helene Berinsky

PUBLISHER'S NOTE
Neither the publisher nor the authors are engaged in rendering professional advice or services to
the individual reader. The ideas, procedures, and suggestions contained in this book are not in-
tended as a substitute for consulting with your physician. All matters regarding your health require medical supervision. Neither the authors nor the publisher shall be liable or responsible for
any loss or damage allegedly arising from any information or suggestion in this book.

The recipes contained in this book are to be followed exactly as written. Neither the publisher nor
the authors are responsible for your specific health or allegy needs that may require medical supervision. Neither the publisher nor the authors are responsible for any adverse reactions to the recipes contained in this book.

From Frank:
To my family, my anchor in storms, real and imagined.

From Maggie:
To my husband Al, the real chef in the family.

ACKNOWLEDGMENTS

There are many, many people who have made contributions to this work of love. We would like to give great thanks to Shannon Marven for her tenacity to get it through the channels for publication, to Jan Miller for her continuous support, and to Madeleine Morel for helping us get the pieces to work together. Carolyn Carlson, my editor at Penguin, always seems to magnify what seems like a pig's ear into something truly remarkable with her creative mind. We would especially like to thank the many wonderful organizations that have come forth with the recipes that fit our nutritional requirements and offered new taste discoveries for specific desired mood changes.

The book probably would not have happened without the lady who inspired us with her courage and passion on *The Dr. Phil Show* with a chocolate addiction and a heart of passion for a better, healthier life, Andrea Laudate. As part of her new plan, she contributed the numerous personal recipes (without chocolate) that taste good and are good for you.

Our family support systems have always been the backbone of any project, and we'd like to express our appreciation of Susan (Frank's wife) and Al (Maggie's husband) for their love and support during the writing of this cookbook.

CONTENTS

INTRODUCTION

If you picked up this book, chances are you are one of the millions of Americans who are excited by the growing body of research that tells us that food can dramatically affect our brains . . . not just how we think on a day-to-day basis, but whether or not we'll retain sharp powers of recall, creativity, and alertness well into our golden years.

As you'll find out, many scientists believe that certain foods contain a wealth of powerful natural substances, from antioxidants to phytochemicals to hormones, that are the secret to brain fitness and optimum mental performance. With this cookbook as your guide, incorporating these foods into your weekly menus has never been simpler—or more delicious. Whether your concern is being more creative, getting your kids to be more attentive, or soothing the stress of long, weary days, the foods and nutrition strategies we discuss here are key.

By the way, "we" are a psychologist and a nutrition writer with many years in our fields, and a special interest in how food affects behavior—and it does, enormously. We know, for example, that people are more focused when their brains are producing brain chemicals called dopamine and norepinephrine, while serotonin, another brain chemical, is associated with calmness and good mood. How does nutrition help? Foods that enhance levels of serotonin in the brain are high in carbohydrates. Cereals, pasta, and bread, for example, can help you reduce anxiety because they step up the production of serotonin. This also explains why some people feel like taking a nap after a lunch of spaghetti, since serotonin can also make you feel sleepy.

What if you need to feel alert and wide awake? Can food pep you up? Absolutely. Simply eat a meal rich in protein such as fish or chicken and watch your powers of concentration magnify. Eating protein-rich foods blocks the production of serotonin, boosting alertness, and it even increases levels of dopamine and norepinephrine, another factor that makes you more alert.

Other natural substances in foods include vitamins, minerals, antioxidants, phytochemicals, and more. Nutrients like vitamin C and folic acid help defeat depression. The minerals iron and boron improve attention, memory, and learning. Antioxidants and phytochemicals protect against brain diseases such as Alzheimer's disease. Certain fats enhance memory and other workings of brain function. There's no end to the good that the right food does for the health of your brain, as well as for your behavior and mood.

Clearly food has the power to both destroy and heal the brain. Just as a nutrient-poor diet can strip the brain of the ability to think and feel appropriately, a nutrient-rich diet can help the brain respond in a positive way to all sorts of psychological crises. Food is one of the most powerful prescriptions you have for maximizing your brain power. By simply eating the right foods, you can control your mind, mood, and memory. However, little of this information has been available to apply to everyday life, until now.

Right now you're probably wondering: Is there a way to naturally jump-start your day? Can you easily fix dinners high in brain-building omega-3 fatty acids? Can you prepare meals that will help your kids do better in school? Can you get your family to eat this stuff? Is there a way to eat to help you with the psychological challenges that inevitably come your way?

The answer to all of those questions, and more, is yes. With delicious recipes from around the country, this book shows you how to easily prepare foods that have been proved in research to build brain power, put an end to stress and blue moods, expand your powers of recall, help relieve pain, boost your intelligence and creativity, and even revitalize your sex life.

Some of you will pick up this cookbook because you love reading recipes. Others, who love to cook and try new dishes, will flip through the pages looking for inspiration. Still others will turn to this book hoping to find strategies for improving brain power. We believe every one of you will find what you are looking for.

That said, let us tell you a little bit about how this book is organized. For starters, it is not organized like a normal cookbook, with chapters focusing on types of dishes (appetizers, main dishes, desserts, and so forth). Instead, we've organized it around psychological issues. Let's say, for instance, you want help on how to reduce your anxiety level. You'd flip over to Chapter Two and read up on "Foods That Soothe Stress and Anxiety." Or maybe your sex life needs jazzing up. Check out what we have to say in Chapter Eleven on "Aphrodisiac Foods." Once you get to the chapter you're personally interested in, you'll find twenty or more recipes, grouped into "Starters and Other Delights," "Smart Side Dishes," "Brain Power Entrées," and "Energizing Desserts." This cookbook is an amalgam of different tastes, too, from American home cooking to ethnic and international dishes, so there's lots of variety and you'll never get bored with any of it. As a bonus, each chapter has specific psychological advice in sections called "Smart Tips" to help you deal with life's many hills and valleys.

Eating is undeniably one of the great pleasures in life. Your motivation to build better brain fitness and mental performance will be greater when you enjoy your food, which is why these delicious recipes give you a tremendous advantage. Yes, they're healthy, too, but healthy cooking does not mean bland or boring— neither flavor nor taste are sacrificed. Trust us, you'll enjoy what we've cooked up here, and so will your family.

Each recipe has been included to help you tackle some of your most pressing psychological issues, but without skimping on the flavors you enjoy. Many of these recipes can be prepared ahead of time and popped in the oven or microwave when you are ready for your next meal. Preparing the recipes usually requires no special equipment, either; everything you need probably is right in your kitchen now.

Many of the recipes in this cookbook have been gathered from trade associations and companies that have graciously lent their permission to use them. Others come from government sources that offer a feast of health dishes. Some are treasured recipes from friends, or are versions that we have adapted to make the most of brain-healing foods. Whatever their source, we're thrilled to share their culinary magic with you. There's more where these came from, too. Be sure to consult the "Resources" section at the back of the book, where you'll find a listing of these organizations and their Web sites, all filled with more great recipes.

There is no limit to the difference healthy, wholesome, and delicious food can make in your life, and we hope you discover its healing gifts with this cookbook. Enjoy these foods and, with them, the new miracles they bring.

—*Dr. Frank Lawlis*
—*Dr. Maggie Greenwood-Robinson*
Dallas, Texas

ONE

※

Brain-Energizing Foods

Just as a car needs gas to run, or your muscles need carbohydrates to move, your brain requires energy to perform its chores, from thinking to remembering to processing the innumerable pieces of data that come its way. But all too often the brain gets short-changed on its energy needs, and we experience mental slumps that make us feel anything but productive. The resulting energy dip can jeopardize your drive, creativity, and impetus to get anything done. This "brain drain" is one of the chief complaints we hear from people, whether they are busy executives, stay-at-home moms, or anyone who is juggling the demands of a busy lifestyle.

But you don't have to succumb to brain drain. Some very minor, easy-to-make changes in your daily diet can have an enormous impact on your mental capabilities, alertness, productivity, and more. With that in mind, we offer a rundown of foods, strategies, and recipes that will keep your mind running at peak performance throughout the day.

Eat Breakfast

Your mom and grandmother were right: Breakfast is a meal you must never miss. Research tells us that people who make a habit of eating breakfast can do more work, are able to maintain their mental efficiency, have faster reaction times, think better, and stay in a more positive frame of mind.

When you get up in the morning, you've been on a fast for about eight to twelve hours. During that time, your body has been using glucose (blood sugar) for energy, and by morning it needs to be restored. The best breakfast for boosting brain power includes natural carbohydrates such as oatmeal, whole grain breads, and other whole grains; protein such as eggs; and some fat. Protein and fat are digested more slowly and thus help your blood sugar stay circulating longer. At breakfast, avoid processed sugar in the form of sugar-laden cereals, pastries, and doughnuts. They cause your blood sugar to spike, then crash to low levels, which leads to physical and mental fatigue. A good brain-boosting breakfast would include a piece of fresh fruit, two cooked eggs, a piece of whole wheat toast with a pat of butter, and a cup of coffee.

Enjoy Protein

For laser-sharp thinking through the day, be sure to eat lean protein at every meal. Protein is essential for physical and mental performance. It builds and repairs tissues, and it contains an amino acid called tyrosine, which promotes clear thinking. Levels of two important neurotransmitters—dopamine and norepinephrine—are increased by eating protein-rich foods. Found in every nook and cranny in the brain, dopamine's chief function is to initiate normal muscle movement, but it also influences attention and the ability to concentrate. As one of the brain's "alert" neurotransmitters, norepinephrine prepares you for action in threatening situations. It also heightens your ability to concentrate.

All proteins are valuable to your brain, but there are two in particular that will keep your brain energized: eggs and yogurt. Eggs are a treasure trove of choline, an essential nutrient for making the brain chemical acetylcholine, required for normal brain function. Enough choline in your brain helps prevent cloudy thinking. Eggs are such an excellent source of choline that you'll want to consider eating three or four a week as part of a brain-energizing diet. Get your kids in the habit of eating eggs, too. One research study found that college students who ate two boiled eggs for breakfast had 10 to 20 percent higher test scores.

Yogurt, an all-around great health food, confers some of the same benefits. In a Tufts University study, students solved math problems in record time after snacking on yogurt rather than drinking a diet soft drink. Yogurt is made up of both protein and carbohydrate, a power-packed combo of nutrients that provides an even release of energy for mental and physical performance. It is also loaded with vitamin D and B vitamins, all nutrients that power up the brain.

Have a Low-Carb Lunch

What you eat at midday has an impact on your mental performance for the rest of the day. The best lunch for reenergizing your brain is one that is low in carbohydrates and high in protein.

Carbs, while nutritious, can make you feel sluggish afterward, whereas protein helps you keep your mental edge. What we suggest is that you enjoy a salad topped with tuna or chicken at lunch, and skip any bread or pasta. You'll be surprised at your mental pep the rest of the afternoon. A number of the main dish salads that follow help fill this bill. At dinner, welcome some carbs back into your meal. Remember, they provide glucose, and glucose is used by the brain to create a neurotransmitter called serotonin. A good supply of serotonin will help you sleep better and get the rest you require for the next day of vigorous mental demands.

Load Up on Fruits and Veggies

Fruits and vegetables are loaded with all sorts of health-boosting nutrients, but the reason they prevent brain drain has to do with one nutrient in particular: potassium. Potassium serves the body in many ways. It assists the nerves in sending messages, helps digestive enzymes do their work, ensures proper muscle functioning (including that of the heart), regulates water balance, and releases energy from protein, carbohydrates, and fats. Potassium also helps prevent mental fatigue.

We can't forget to remind you that fruits and vegetables are brimming with antioxidants, too. The brain consumes more oxygen than any other organ in the body, and thus is highly vulnerable to oxidation, a tissue-damaging process that occurs when oxygen reacts with fat. The by-products of this reaction are free radicals, which attack cell membranes and ultimately lead to disease. Antioxidants, available from food and made naturally by the body, neutralize free radicals and interrupt this process. Several of the recipes in this chapter are packed with high-antioxidant foods such as Concord grape juice, pomegranate juice, citrus fruits, squash, and green leafy vegetables.

Pump Up Your Iron

Many of the foods we recommend here for mental alertness— yogurt; lean proteins such as chicken, tuna, or lean red meat; and green leafy vegetables—are also naturally high in the mineral iron. Iron helps your brain access the oxygen it needs for peak functioning. It is also deposited in a part of your brain that stimulates and maintains alertness. When you eat vitamin C–rich foods such as citrus fruits or peppers, your body better absorbs iron. Eating iron-rich foods is an easy way to help stay mentally focused.

On days when you're on the go—picking up kids, solving problems at work, or giving a presentation—and you want to avoid mental slumps, try some of the recipes in this chapter, which include foods that can help fuel your brain and provide all-day stamina when you need it. Enjoy!

SMART TIPS ✸ MORE BRAIN ENERGIZERS

- **DRINK UP:** To maintain peak mental capacity, drink eight to ten glasses of pure water every day. This will prevent dehydration or water deficiency. Even if you're mildly dehydrated, your mental performance will suffer. Thus, to think, we need to drink plenty of water!

continued

- **AVOID BRAIN-DRAINING DRUGS:** These include alcohol, antihistamines, blood pressure medications, and some antidepressants—all of which tend to cloud thinking and impair memory.

- **MOVE YOUR BODY, ACTIVATE YOUR BRAIN:** What's good for your body is good for your brain—and that includes regular exercise. Exercise boosts the flow of oxygenated blood to your brain. In addition, exercise boosts reaction time and enhances the synthesis of neurotransmitters, which are required for the rapid transmission of messages throughout the body.

HOW TO GET YOUR KIDS TO EAT THE RIGHT STUFF

- Gradually eliminate some snack foods by providing your kids with better replacement food choices, such as fruits instead of candy or frozen yogurt instead of ice cream.

- Invite your kids to help you prepare meals. This can create warm, lasting childhood memories for them. In the process of fixing meals, they can learn about various food groups and the importance of each.

- Emphasize the qualities of foods that will appeal to your child. For example: It will help you do better in sports, make a good grade on your test, grow up to be strong, make your hair look pretty, or feel happy when you go to school.

- Try a "one bite" rule in your household, meaning that your children only have to taste a food for a single bite. If they don't like it, leave it alone for that meal. This gives your children some control over what they will or will not eat. Tastes mature, so your kids may come to like something they previously disliked. But for that to happen, you have to at least introduce the foods so their preferences can expand over time.

- Model healthy eating. Your kids watch what you do, so be a positive role model by eating nutritiously.

- Reinforce good eating habits by congratulating your children for exploring new foods.

STARTERS AND OTHER DELIGHTS

Pomegranate Smoothie

1 banana
2 cups nonfat vanilla yogurt
1 cup pomegranate juice
1 tablespoon sugar (optional)

Peel the banana and wrap in plastic wrap. Freeze for 3 hours, or until frozen. Unwrap the banana, break it into chunks, and place in a blender with the yogurt and juice. Cover and blend until smooth; pour into 4 glasses and serve immediately. Serving tip: Before serving, wet the edges of the glasses and dip them into sugar for a decorative edge.

Makes 4 servings

Recipe courtesy of Dairy Management Inc.

Yogurt Deviled Eggs

6 hard-cooked eggs, peeled
¼ cup lowfat plain yogurt
1 teaspoon dried minced onion
1 teaspoon parsley flakes or freeze-dried chives
1 teaspoon fresh lemon juice
¾ teaspoon prepared mustard
¼ teaspoon salt (optional)
¼ teaspoon Worcestershire sauce
⅛ teaspoon black pepper
Dash of paprika

Cut the eggs in half lengthwise. Remove the yolks and set the whites aside. In a small bowl, mash the yolks with fork. Add the yogurt, onion, parsley, lemon juice, mustard, salt, if using, the Worcestershire sauce, pepper, and paprika and stir until well blended. Using a spoon or pastry bag, fill the whites, using about 1 tablespoon of the yolk mixture for each egg half.

Makes 12 appetizer servings

Recipe courtesy of the American Egg Board

Zesty Vegetable Egg Spread

1 cup bottled reduced-fat ranch dressing
4 ounces Neufchâtel cheese, softened
2 tablespoons fresh lemon juice
4 hard-cooked eggs, peeled and chopped
2 tablespoons grated carrot

2 tablespoons finely chopped green onions with tops
2 tablespoons finely chopped mushroom, any type
2 tablespoons finely chopped radish

In a medium bowl, combine the dressing, cheese, and lemon juice and stir until smooth and creamy. Stir in the remaining ingredients. Cover and refrigerate to blend the flavors. Serve as a spread with crackers or as a dip for fresh vegetables.

Yields approximately 1½ cups

Recipe courtesy of the American Egg Board

Huevos Rancheros with Fresh Salsa

Four 6-inch corn tortillas
½ tablespoon vegetable oil
Nonstick cooking spray
4 medium egg whites
4 medium whole eggs
⅛ teaspoon ground black pepper
4 tablespoons shredded cheddar or Monterey Jack cheese
2 cups prepared salsa

Preheat the oven to 450°F. Lightly brush the tortillas on both sides with oil and place on a baking sheet. Bake for 5 to 10 minutes, until the tortillas are crisp on the edges and starting to brown. Remove from the oven and set aside.

Spray a large skillet with cooking spray and place over medium heat. Drop the egg whites into the skillet, then break the whole eggs over the whites to make 4 separate servings. Cook for 2 to 3 minutes on each side, until the eggs are cooked.

Place 1 egg on each tortilla shell, top each with 1 tablespoon of the cheese, and sprinkle with black pepper. Place under the broiler for about 2 minutes, or until the cheese is melted. Spoon ½ cup fresh salsa around the edge of each shell.

Makes 4 to 6 servings

Source: Food Stamp Nutrition Connection

Cranberry Avocado Salsa

1 yellow bell pepper
One 12-ounce bag (3 cups) fresh or frozen cranberries
½ cup sugar
¼ cup orange juice
1 jalapeño chile, seeded and chopped
1 tablespoon grated orange zest
2 ripe Hass avocados, peeled, pitted, and diced
¼ cup chopped fresh cilantro
Salt and black pepper

Char the bell pepper over a gas flame or in the broiler, turning with tongs, until the skin has blackened on all sides. Place the charred pepper in a paper bag to steam off the skin for about 10 minutes. Peel, seed, and chop the bell pepper.

Combine the cranberries, sugar, and orange juice in a food processor. Pulse the mixture to coarsely chop the cranberries. Transfer to a medium bowl. Add the bell pepper, jalapeño, and orange zest. (The salsa can be prepared up to this point 1 day ahead. Cover and refrigerate until ready to serve.) Stir the avocado and cilantro into the mixture. Season with salt and pepper to taste. Serve with whole wheat crackers or tortilla chips.

Makes 3½ cups

Recipe courtesy of the Cape Cod Cranberry Growers' Association

SMART SIDE DISHES

Beet and Tomato Casserole

2½ cups sliced canned beets, drained
2½ cups canned tomatoes
½ cup grated mozzarella cheese
Salt and black pepper
2 cups breadcrumbs
2 tablespoons unsalted butter

Preheat the oven to 350°F.

Arrange half of the beets in the bottom of a greased 9×13-inch baking dish. Make a second layer with half the tomatoes, then half the cheese. Sprinkle with salt and pepper, if needed. Top with half the breadcrumbs, then dot with half of the butter. Repeat the layering with the rest of the ingredients. Bake for 20 minutes, or until browned on top. Serve immediately.

Makes 6 servings

Recipe courtesy of the Pioneer Valley Growers Association

Italian Vegetable Bake

One 28-ounce can whole tomatoes
1 medium onion, sliced
½ pound fresh green beans, sliced

½ pound fresh okra, cut into ½-inch pieces, or half of
  a 10-ounce package frozen okra
¾ cup finely chopped green bell pepper
2 tablespoons fresh lemon juice
1 teaspoon chopped fresh basil, or 1 teaspoon dried basil,
  crushed
1½ teaspoons chopped fresh oregano leaves, or ½ teaspoon dried
  oregano, crushed
3 medium (7-inch-long) zucchinis, cut into 1-inch cubes
1 medium eggplant, peeled and cut into 1-inch cubes
2 tablespoons grated Parmesan cheese

Preheat the oven to 325°F.

Drain the tomatoes, reserving the juices, and coarsely chop.
Combine the tomatoes and reserved liquid, the onion, green
beans, okra, green pepper, lemon juice, basil, and oregano.
Cover with foil and bake in a 9×13-inch baking dish for 15
minutes. Remove the foil and stir in the zucchini and eggplant.
Cover again and bake for 60 to 70 minutes, until the vegetables
are tender, stirring occasionally. Just before serving, sprinkle the
top with the cheese.

Makes eight 1-cup servings

Source: U.S. Department of Health and Human Services

Plum Salad

¼ cup pine nuts
1 tablespoon red wine vinegar
4 tablespoons orange juice

1½ teaspoons grated orange zest
4 tablespoons olive oil
Salt and black pepper
1 small head radicchio (about 5 ounces), torn into 2-inch pieces
3 large handfuls arugula (about 5 ounces)
2 endives
3 oranges, sectioned
½ cup (about 3 ounces) dried plums, pitted and halved

Place the pine nuts in a dry skillet placed over medium heat. Shaking the pan constantly, cook the pine nuts until light golden, 1 to 2 minutes. Remove from the heat and set aside to cool.

In a medium bowl, whisk together the vinegar, orange juice, orange zest, and oil. Season with salt and pepper to taste.

In a large bowl, toss the radicchio and arugula together. Cut the tip off the endive on a diagonal. Continue to turn and cut the endive into diagonal pieces. Add to the salad, along with the oranges and dried plums. Add the vinaigrette and toss. Garnish the salad with the toasted pine nuts and serve immediately.

Makes 4 servings

Recipe courtesy of the California Dried Plum Board

Glazed Carrots with Dried Plums

1 pound (about 6 medium) carrots, cut into 2-inch pieces,
    or baby carrots
½ cup orange juice
1 tablespoon honey

2 teaspoons prepared yellow mustard
⅛ teaspoon black pepper
1 cup (about 6 ounces) pitted dried plums, halved
1 tablespoon unsalted butter
Salt
2 tablespoons chopped fresh parsley (optional)

Place the carrots in a large skillet with water to cover. Place over high heat and bring to a boil. Reduce the heat to medium and cook for about 10 minutes, or until crisp-tender; drain and return to the skillet. Meanwhile, in a small bowl, whisk together the orange juice, honey, mustard, and pepper. Add the dried plums, butter, and orange juice mixture to the carrots. Bring to a simmer, then reduce the heat to low, cover, and cook for 5 to 10 minutes, stirring occasionally, until the sauce thickens slightly and is reduced by half. Season with salt to taste. Garnish with the parsley, if using.

Makes 4 servings

Recipe courtesy of the California Dried Plum Board

Waldorf Salad

2 crisp red-skinned apples, such as Jonagold or Red Delicious
    (to make 3 cups chopped)
2 tablespoons fresh lemon juice
2 ribs celery, diced (about ½ cup)
2 tablespoons chopped toasted walnuts
¼ cup lowfat mayonnaise dressing
4 cups romaine lettuce, torn into bite-size pieces
¼ cup raisins

Cut the apples into quarters, core them, then cut into ¾-inch pieces. Place in a large bowl and toss with the lemon juice. Add the celery, walnuts, and mayonnaise dressing and mix thoroughly. Arrange the lettuce on 4 plates or in salad bowls. Scoop the apple mixture onto each salad and scatter the raisins over the top.

Makes 4 servings

Source: U.S. Department of Health and Human Services

Sunshine Salad

5 cups packed spinach leaves
½ red onion, sliced thin
½ red bell pepper, sliced
1 medium cucumber, sliced
2 oranges, peeled and chopped into bite-size pieces
½ cup bottled reduced-fat vinaigrette dressing

Toss all the ingredients except the dressing together in a large bowl. Add the dressing and toss again. Serve immediately.

Makes 4 servings

Source: U.S. Department of Health and Human Services

BRAIN POWER ENTRÉES

Vegetable and Rice Quiche

6 medium eggs
2 cups cooked and cooled brown rice (⅔ cup raw)
One 10-ounce package frozen chopped broccoli

⅓ cup chopped green bell pepper
⅓ cup chopped green onions with tops
1 clove garlic, minced
¾ cup (about 3 ounces) shredded reduced-fat cheddar cheese
One 2-ounce jar drained sliced pimientos
One 2-ounce can drained sliced mushrooms
½ cup skim or lowfat milk

Preheat the oven to 375°F.

In a medium bowl, beat 1 of the eggs. Add the rice and stir until well blended. Press the mixture onto the bottom and up the sides of a lightly greased 9-inch pie plate or shallow baking dish. Set aside.

In a nonstick skillet, combine the broccoli, bell pepper, green onions, and garlic. Place over medium heat, cover, and cook, stirring occasionally, until the broccoli is thawed, about 5 minutes. Set aside to cool slightly. Stir in the cheese, pimientos, and mushrooms. Spoon into the prepared crust.

In a large bowl, beat together remaining 5 eggs and the milk until well blended. Pour over the vegetables and place in the oven. Bake for 35 to 45 minutes, until a knife inserted near the center comes out clean.

Makes 6 servings

Recipe courtesy of the American Egg Board

Southwest Salad

1 pound lean ground beef
½ cup chopped onions

1 tablespoon chili powder
2 teaspoons ground cumin
1 cup canned red kidney beans, drained
One 15-ounce can chickpeas, drained
1 medium tomato, diced
2 cups shredded lettuce
½ cup shredded cheddar cheese

In a large skillet over medium-high heat, cook the ground beef and onions until the beef is no longer pink. Drain. Stir the chili powder and cumin into the beef mixture, and cook for 1 minute. Add the kidney beans, chickpeas, and tomato. Mix gently to combine.

Combine the lettuce and cheese in a large serving bowl. Portion the lettuce and cheese among 4 plates. Divide the beef mixture among the plates.

Makes 4 servings

Source: U.S. Department of Health and Human Services

Simply Spaghetti Squash

1 large spaghetti squash, halved lengthwise and cleaned
About ½ cup water
½ cup olive oil
½ cup balsamic vinegar or red wine vinegar
1 tablespoon Italian seasoning (oregano, rosemary, and thyme)
2 cloves garlic, minced
2 plum tomatoes, chopped
½ cup shredded Parmesan or Romano cheeses, or a combination

Preheat the oven to 350°F.

In a large, shallow baking pan, place the squash halves cut side down. Add water to a depth of ¼ inch. Cover loosely with foil, place in the oven, and bake for 20 minutes.

Meanwhile, in a small bowl or measuring cup, whisk together the oil, vinegar, Italian seasoning, and garlic. Add the tomatoes. Set the dressing aside.

Remove the squash from the oven and remove the foil (it can be reused). Slice ½ inch off the top of each half so that the squash won't wobble when placed cut side up on a plate.

Take a fork and fluff the squash so that it becomes the spaghetti it is named for. Alternative method: After fluffing and separating the squash, spoon it out onto a plate.

Whisk the dressing and pour it over the squash. Sprinkle with the cheese and serve.

Makes 4 to 6 servings

Recipe courtesy of Andrea Laudate

Lemon Chicken

2 whole boneless chicken breasts
Salt
½ cup cornstarch
⅓ cup olive oil
2 cups coarsely shredded iceberg lettuce
4 or 5 very thin lemon slices

SAUCE
3 tablespoons fresh lemon juice
3 tablespoons sugar
1½ teaspoons light soy sauce

1 teaspoon sesame oil
1 tablespoon olive oil
¼ teaspoon salt
⅓ cup low-sodium chicken broth
2 tablespoons water
2½ teaspoons cornstarch

Score the chicken breasts so they don't curl up and season lightly with salt. Pat the ½ cup cornstarch over both sides of the breasts. Let stand a few moments and pat it again so the corn-starch sticks.

Heat the ⅓ cup oil in a large skillet over medium heat. Add the chicken breasts and cook for 10 to 12 minutes on each side, until lightly browned and cooked through

While you brown the chicken breasts, combine the sauce ingredients in a medium saucepan over medium heat. Bring to a simmer and cook until thickened, adding cornstarch as needed.

Arrange lettuce on a platter and place the chicken on top. Pour the sauce over the chicken. Arrange the lemon slices on top of the chicken and serve.

Makes 2 servings

Source: Food Stamp Nutrition Connection

Ground Chicken Stir-Fry

1½ teaspoons peanut or vegetable oil
1 to 2 dried hot chiles (optional)
5 ounces ground lean chicken
1 cup sliced onions
1 cup sliced mushrooms

1 cup red bell pepper strips
1 cup broccoli florets
1 clove garlic, minced
1 teaspoon minced fresh ginger
1 cup low-sodium chicken broth
1 teaspoon cornstarch
½ teaspoon toasted sesame oil

Heat the peanut oil in a 9-inch skillet or wok over medium-high heat. Add the chiles, if using, and cook for 30 seconds. Using a slotted spoon, remove and discard the chiles. Raise the heat to high; add the chicken, onions, mushrooms, bell pepper, broccoli, garlic, and ginger to the skillet; and cook for 3 minutes, or until chicken is no longer pink, stirring frequently.

In a small bowl, combine the broth, cornstarch, and sesame oil, stirring to dissolve the cornstarch. Stir into the chicken-vegetable mixture and cook, stirring constantly, until the mixture comes to a boil. Reduce the heat to low and simmer for about 5 minutes, or until thoroughly heated.

Makes 2 servings

Recipe Courtesy of Andrea Laudate

Crispy Oven-Fried Chicken

1 teaspoon vegetable oil
½ cup skim milk or buttermilk
1 teaspoon poultry seasoning
1 cup crumbled cornflakes
1½ tablespoons onion powder
1½ tablespoons garlic powder

2 teaspoons black pepper
2 teaspoons crushed red chile flakes
1 teaspoon ground ginger
8 pieces skinless chicken (4 breasts and drumsticks)
Dash of paprika

In a medium bowl, combine the milk with ½ teaspoon of the poultry seasoning. In a heavy-duty zip-top bag, combine the cornflake crumbs with the remaining poultry seasoning, the onion powder, garlic powder, black pepper, chile flakes, and ginger.

Wash the chicken and pat dry with paper towels. Dip the chicken into the milk, shake to remove excess, then quickly shake the chicken in the bag with the cornflake crumbs. Seal the bag and refrigerate for 1 hour.

Preheat the oven to 350°F. Coat a baking pan with the oil. Remove the chicken from the plastic bag and sprinkle lightly with paprika. Place the chicken pieces on the baking pan. Cover with foil and bake for 40 minutes. Remove the foil and bake for an additional 30 to 40 minutes, until the meat can be easily pulled away from the bone with a fork. The drumsticks may require less baking time than the breasts. Do not turn the chicken while it bakes. The cornflake crumbs will form a crispy coating. Cut the chicken breasts in half and serve.

Makes 4 to 6 servings

Source: Food Stamp Nutrition Connection

Mouthwatering Oven-Fried Fish

1 tablespoon vegetable oil
6 fish fillets, 6 to 8 ounces each (perch, tilapia, cod, any whitefish)

1 tablespoon fresh lemon juice
1 cup skim milk or buttermilk
2 drops hot pepper sauce
1 teaspoon minced garlic
½ cup crumbled cornflakes, or breadcrumbs
¼ teaspoon ground white pepper
¼ teaspoon salt
¼ teaspoon onion powder
1 lemon, cut into 6 wedges

Preheat the oven to 475°F. Coat a large baking dish with the oil.

Wipe the fish fillets with the lemon juice and pat dry. In a medium bowl, combine the milk, hot pepper sauce, and garlic. On a large plate, combine the cornflake crumbs, pepper, salt, and onion powder. Place the fish fillets in the milk and let sit briefly. Remove and coat fillets on both sides with the seasoned crumbs. Let stand briefly, until the coating sticks to each side of the fish.

Arrange the fish fillets on the baking dish and bake for 20 minutes on the middle rack without turning, or until fish flakes easily with a fork. Remove from the oven and serve immediately with the lemon slices.

Makes 6 servings

Source: U.S. Department of Health and Human Services

Tuna Salad

Two 6-ounce cans water packed tuna
½ cup chopped celery

⅓ *cup chopped green onions*
6½ *tablespoons reduced-fat mayonnaise*

Place the tuna in a strainer and break it apart with a fork. Rinse the tuna and drain for 5 minutes. Place the tuna in a medium bowl and add the celery, green onions, and mayonnaise. Mix well.

Makes 4 servings

Source: U.S. Department of Health and Human Services

ENERGIZING DESSERTS

Lemon Pudding Custard

Nonstick cooking spray
4 large eggs
½ *cup sugar*
3 tablespoons fresh lemon juice
2 teaspoons grated lemon zest
1½ *teaspoons vanilla extract*
¼ *teaspoon salt (optional)*
3 cups skim or lowfat milk, heated until very hot
Sliced fresh strawberries, to garnish
Jam, jelly, or fruit preserves, to garnish
Lemon peel strips, to garnish (optional)
Fresh mint leaves, to garnish (optional)

Preheat the oven to 350°F. Coat six 6-ounce custard cups with cooking spray and place in a large baking pan.

In a medium bowl, beat together the eggs, sugar, lemon juice, lemon zest, vanilla, and salt, if using, until well blended. Stir in the milk. Pour the egg mixture into the custard cups. Place the pan in the oven and pour *very* hot water into the pan to within ½ inch of the top of the custards.

Bake until a knife inserted near the center comes out clean, 25 to 30 minutes. Remove the custards promptly from the pan. Cool on a wire rack for 5 to 10 minutes. Serve warm or chilled. Invert onto individual plates. Arrange sliced strawberries around each custard and spoon jam on top. Garnish with lemon peel strips and mint leaves, if using.

Makes 6 servings

Recipe courtesy of the American Egg Board

Frosty Blueberry Custard

2 cups fresh or frozen blueberries
4 large eggs
2 cups buttermilk
½ cup sugar
1½ tablespoons fresh lemon juice
2 envelopes unflavored gelatin
1 cup nonfat lemon yogurt (optional)

Set aside 8 blueberries for garnish, if desired. Place the remaining blueberries in a blender and set aside.

In a medium saucepan, beat together the eggs, buttermilk, sugar, and lemon juice until blended. Sprinkle with the gelatin and let stand for 1 minute. Place over low heat and cook, stirring constantly, until the mixture just coats a metal spoon with a thin film and reaches 160°F. Pour over the berries in the blender container and blend at high speed until well blended, about 30 seconds.

Pour into a 5-cup mold. Cover directly with plastic and chill until set, several hours or overnight. To serve, unmold on a platter and top with the yogurt and reserved berries, if using.

Makes 8 servings

Recipe courtesy of the American Egg Board

Citrus Grape Sherbert

½ *gallon lemon sherbert*
6 *cups Concord grape juice*
2 *cups Concord grape jam or jelly*
¼ *cup grated lemon zest*

Let the sherbert soften slightly in the refrigerator. Spoon into a blender or food processor and add the Concord grape juice, Concord grape jam, and lemon zest. Blend on low speed until thoroughly mixed. Do not let sherbert melt completely. Pour into a large freezer container and freeze until firm.

Makes 8 servings

Recipe courtesy of the Concord Grape Association

Orange and Dried Plum Compote

6 *seedless oranges*
½ *cup pitted dried plums (about 3 ounces), quartered lengthwise*
½ *cup water*
⅓ *cup sugar*

1 tablespoon rosewater
¼ cup pomegranate seeds, dried cranberries, or pistachios
¼ cup shredded mint leaves
Pinch of ground cardamom
Pinch of ground cinnamon

With a sharp knife, cut away the peel of the oranges, making sure to remove all white pith. Cut the oranges across into ½-inch rounds. Place the oranges and dried plums in a large bowl. In a small saucepan over medium heat, combine the water and sugar. Bring to a simmer and simmer just until the sugar dissolves. Remove from the heat, cool, and add the rosewater. Pour the mixture over the oranges and dried plums. Cover and refrigerate at least 20 minutes; the compote may be prepared to this point up to 1 day ahead.

To serve, arrange the oranges and dried plums in a shallow bowl or deep platter and pour the liquid over them. Top with the pomegranate seeds and mint and sprinkle with the cardamom and cinnamon.

Makes 6 servings

Recipe courtesy of the California Dried Plum Board

Dutch Apple Yogurt Dessert

½ cup nonfat plain yogurt
½ cup unsweetened applesauce
1 tablespoon seedless raisins
1 teaspoon brown sugar
⅛ teaspoon ground cinnamon
1 tablespoon chopped walnuts or pecans or crunchy cereal

Combine the yogurt, applesauce, raisins, brown sugar, and cinnamon in a small bowl. Cover and refrigerate until chilled. Spoon into serving bowls and top with the nuts.

Makes 2 servings

Source: Food Stamp Nutrition Connection

TWO

※

Foods That Soothe
Stress and Anxiety

Blowing a sales call, missing deadlines, failing a test, getting laid off, working too hard, losing a loved one—these are just a few of the things in life that trigger stress and, with it, emotions of frustration, anxiety, even depression. Medical experts estimate that stress accounts for more than 90 percent of all illnesses and trips to the doctor, for an array of ailments, from skin problems to headaches to infections triggered by the assault of stress on the immune system. Chronic stress also robs your body of nutrients such as vitamin C, vitamin B complex, and protein.

So what's a stressed-out body to do? One of the most overlooked strategies of combating stress is nutrition, and one of the best places to start lightening your load is in your kitchen. You can manipulate your brain chemistry to stay calm by what you put on your plate. Food can definitely be a "mood drug," and many "calming" foods are common, everyday staples.

At my clinic in Lewisville, Texas, we often analyze the diets of children and teenagers who come to us for various behavioral problems, including stress-related issues, and we've seen some astounding changes in behavior—for the better—when a few adjustments are made in a kid's diet.

A child who comes to mind is Maria, a bright-eyed twelve-year-old, who had become a major thorn in her teacher's side. Several times a week she was sent to the principal's office for acting like the "class clown" and disrupting the classroom, especially during math instruction. When we questioned Maria, she confessed that math was scary to her, and she felt frustrated when she couldn't "get it." The more anxious she got, the less she focused on learning the lessons. Like most kids these days, Maria subsisted on a diet laced with refined sugar and refined carbohydrates including white flour, sugary breakfast cereals, and high-fructose corn syrup (found in soft drinks, juice drinks, and many processed foods). She was taking in so much sugar that it was showing up in her behavior in the form of anxiety and irritability. Not only that, she was eating too many processed foods and fast foods, many filled with coloring agents, which have been implicated in triggering stress-related conditions such as hypersensitivity. It took some doing, and a commitment from her mother, but we got her to bring "low-stress foods" to school for lunch and snacks. Out went the french fries and soft drinks; in came fresh and dried fruits, unsalted nuts, sandwiches made with high-fiber bread, and yogurt. The transformation in Maria's behavior and school performance was remarkable: In a matter of weeks, Maria was paying attention to lessons, and her math grades improved.

Just about anyone—children or adults—can eat their way to calm, and here's how to do it:

Limit Caffeine

Certainly caffeinated foods such as coffee or tea have brain-boosting powers (like greater alertness and creativity), but they're counterproductive if you're prone to stress. Caffeine elevates stress hormones such as cortisol in the body, and chronically high levels of stress hormones can lead to artery damage, cholesterol buildup, and heart disease; they also can weaken your immune system. Another reason for cutting back on caffeine has to do with an important stress-buster: sleep. Caffeine can interfere with quality sleep, which you need to soothe stress. Like the restart button for your computer, quality sleep is vital for maintaining emotional balance. When you "crash," shut-eye gives your body time to reboot.

Ease Back on Simple Sugars

As a general rule of thumb, it's a good idea, particularly during times of stress, to ease up on simple sugars and no-nutrient junk foods like potato chips, candy, cakes, and ice cream. The elevation in blood sugar and insulin they provide, combined with the already high levels of cortisol in your body, can lead you to eat more and put you at risk of insulin insensitivity and diabetes. Seek healthier comfort foods instead, such as nonfat or lowfat yogurt instead of ice cream; dried vegetable chips or raw veggies instead of potato chips. Also, populate your diet with complex carbohydrates in the form of whole grains; their steady release of sugar both keeps your blood sugar levels steady and induces your brain to churn out more of the feel-good chemical serotonin.

Stress-Busting B Vitamins

The B vitamins have been dubbed "antistress nutrients" because they are often the first deficiencies to develop during periods of stress. As water-soluble vitamins, they are not stored in bodily tissues to any great extent, so deficiencies can develop rather rapidly. Thiamine (vitamin B_1) and riboflavin (vitamin B_2) are particularly important because of their role in energy production. Thiamine helps provide energy to nerve cells by converting fuel from carbohydrates into energy in the form of glucose. Because glucose is the only source of energy for the nervous system, an adequate amount of B_1 means steadier nerves. A deficiency of thiamine can lead to degeneration of the insulation—called the myelin sheath—that protects nerve fibers. As a result, nerves become hypersensitive and irritable and stress heightens. Foods high in thiamine include green peas, spinach, legumes, whole grains, pork, beef, soy foods, and bananas.

Riboflavin (vitamin B_2) also helps release energy from carbohydrates, proteins, and fats. It helps the body produce antistress hormones and is critical to the health of the glandular system, particularly the adrenal glands. Among other functions, the adrenals release hormones crucial to nervous system health. Whole grains, eggs, shellfish, green vegetables, legumes, mushrooms, meat, yogurt, and cheeses are high in riboflavin.

During any type of stress, when enormous amounts of adrenal hormones are pressed into service, the need for pantothenic acid (vitamin B_5) skyrockets. A short supply of it is especially damaging to the adrenal glands, which become enlarged and unable to produce hormones when needed. By sparing adrenal hormones, pantothenic acid prevents the adrenal glands from becoming fatigued. Whole grains, eggs, meats, and legumes are high in pantothenic acid.

Go Bananas

Bananas are one of the rare fruits that help quell anxiety, and we often recommend several bananas a day to patients under stress. That's because bananas are full of magnesium, a mineral depleted by chronic stress, as well as the B vitamins mentioned on page 31. Bananas also help the body produce more serotonin for a greater sense of well-being.

Eat More Fruits and Vegetables

On practically every page of this cookbook, we'll be rooting for fruits and vegetables as mainstays in your diet. Not only do fruits and vegetables keep your gastrointestinal tract working during high-stress periods (and help you avoid constipation), but the nutrients they provide lend an extra layer of protection against chronic stress. Under stress, the body produces more disease-causing free radicals, so it is crucial to provide more antioxidants, which help neutralize free radicals. Antioxidants abound in fresh fruits and vegetables, so be sure you eat plenty every day. One antioxidant in particular, vitamin C, is considered a natural tranquilizer. Citrus fruits and bell peppers are high in vitamin C.

Enjoy Food Cooked with Love

Ancient teachings from cultures the world over have pointed out that the vibration of the cook's feelings affects not only the quality of the food, but the emotional state of those being fed. This is why it is ideal to serve and eat home-cooked meals whenever possible, because food prepared in a restaurant by strangers doesn't have the positive energy of a meal cooked by someone who loves you. When you cook for your friends or family, be in a happy frame of mind because you'll transfer positive emotions to them, and this helps relieve stress or tension. And when you're cooking, focus on the food and make it a settled, conscious event rather than something you're throwing together under pressure. Turn off the TV, and give yourself time to enjoy the simple act of smelling the spices, feeling the textures of the foods, playing with the colors, and having fun. Make meal preparation a happy, relaxed time. Your positive thoughts and feelings will make the meal a true feast.

With these strategies in mind, we introduce you to a collection of recipes that incorporate an array of stress-busting foods.

SMART TIPS ⚫ STRESS BUSTERS

- Pamper yourself—with a massage, a manicure, or a session at a day spa.

- Take mini-time-outs to read or relax.

- Incorporate mind-body exercise, such as yoga or tai chi, into your life.

- Don't bring your work home.   continued

- Become engrossed in a favorite hobby for distraction.

- Take a vacation, even if it is just for a weekend.

- Talk out your problems with a friend or qualified counselor.

- Pursue spiritual activities such as prayer or meditation.

- Take control of your time by making short to-do lists, but don't get frustrated if you fail to complete everything on the list.

- Take steps to resolve whatever is causing the stress. If it is financial, see a financial counselor about creating a better budget; if it's a relationship, try couples therapy.

- Whatever is stressing you out, do not self-medicate with food, alcohol, or drugs.

STARTERS AND OTHER DELIGHTS

Flax-Canola Prairie Bread (Bread Machine)

1¼ cups water
2 tablespoons honey
2 tablespoons canola oil
2 cups bread flour
1 cup whole wheat flour
1½ teaspoons salt
⅓ cup flax seeds
2 tablespoons sunflower seeds
1 tablespoon poppy seeds
2 teaspoons quick-rising instant yeast

Place the ingredients in the bread machine pan in the order recommended by the manufacturer. Select "Whole Wheat Rapid Cycle." Remove the baked bread from the pan and let cool on a wire rack.

Makes 1 loaf

Recipe courtesy of the Northern Canola Growers Association

Fruit and Nut Hot Cereal

3⅓ cups water
⅔ cup instant rolled oats
⅔ cup oat bran
One 6-ounce package diced fruit bits
½ teaspoon salt (optional)
¼ cup coarsely chopped walnuts
Brown sugar, to serve (optional)
Skim milk, to serve (optional)

In a medium saucepan over medium heat, bring the water to boil. Stir in the oats, oat bran, fruit bits, and salt, if using. Bring to a boil and cook for 2 to 5 minutes, stirring frequently. Stir in the walnuts. Serve with brown sugar and skim milk, if using.

Makes 4 servings

Recipe courtesy of the North American Millers' Association

Barley Granola

¾ cup vegetable oil
¾ cup honey

1½ tablespoons vanilla extract

⅓ cup water

½ tablespoon salt

2 cups quick-cooking rolled barley

6 cups quick-cooking rolled oats

1 cup wheat germ

1 cup unsweetened, flaked coconut

⅓ cup brown sugar

1½ cups raisins (optional)

1 cup chopped nuts and seeds (combination of your
   choice of peanuts, almonds, sunflower seeds,
   sesame seeds)

In a medium bowl, whisk together the oil, honey, vanilla, water, and salt until well mixed. In a large bowl, combine the remaining ingredients. Pour the liquid ingredients over the dry and mix well. Spread the mixture ½ inch deep in shallow baking pans. Bake for 30 minutes, then stir and continue baking, stirring every 15 minutes, until golden brown, about 1½ hours total.

Yields approximately 12 cups

Recipe courtesy of the Idaho Barley Commission

Banana Breakfast Shake

2 medium ripe bananas, peeled, quartered, and frozen

1 cup plain yogurt

⅓ cup papaya-orange juice

2 teaspoons honey

Combine the bananas, yogurt, juice, and honey in a blender or food processor and blend until thick and smooth. Pour into 2 glasses and serve immediately.

Makes 2 servings

Recipe courtesy of Maggie Greenwood-Robinson

Refreshing Summer Shake

1½ cups fresh strawberries, blueberries, or peach slices
½ cup skim milk or ¼ cup nonfat dry milk powder mixed with
*   ½ cup water*
¼ cup lowfat vanilla yogurt
4 ice cubes, crushed

Cut the fruit into pieces and mash through a strainer or with a fork. (If using peaches, peel and core first.) Combine the fruit, milk, and yogurt in a blender or food processor and blend until thick and smooth. Add the crushed ice and blend to combine. Pour into 2 glasses and serve immediately.

Makes 2 servings

Source: Bureau of Markets/Farmers' Markets

SMART SIDE DISHES

Chickpea and Pasta Salad

SALAD
3 cups cooked corkscrew pasta, cooled
One 14-ounce can chickpeas, rinsed and drained

½ cup chopped celery
½ cup coarsely shredded carrot
⅓ cup chopped green bell pepper
2 tablespoons finely sliced green onion tops
1 medium tomato, cut into wedges, to garnish

DRESSING
¼ cup vinegar
2 tablespoons reduced-fat mayonnaise
1 tablespoon canola oil
2 teaspoons Dijon-style mustard
¼ teaspoon salt
¼ teaspoon black pepper

In a large bowl, combine the pasta, chickpeas, celery, carrots, green pepper, and green onions. Toss lightly until evenly mixed.

In a medium bowl, whisk together the vinegar, mayonnaise, oil, mustard, salt, and pepper until blended. Pour over the pasta and vegetables and toss until evenly coated. Cover and refrigerate for 2 hours. Serve, garnished with the tomato wedges. The salad will keep for up to 2 days.

Makes 4 servings

Recipe courtesy of the Northern Canola Growers Association

Creole Zucchini

1 tablespoon vegetable oil or olive oil
½ cup chopped onion
½ clove garlic, minced, or a dash of garlic powder
½ cup chopped green bell pepper

1 pound zucchini, sliced
2 medium tomatoes, peeled and chopped
⅛ teaspoon salt
⅛ teaspoon black pepper
2 tablespoons grated Parmesan cheese
2 tablespoons chopped fresh parsley (optional)

In a large sauté pan, heat the oil over medium heat. Add the onion, garlic, and green pepper and sauté until softened, about 5 minutes. Add the zucchini, tomatoes, salt, and pepper. Cover and cook until the zucchini is tender, about 20 minutes. Serve immediately, topped with the cheese and parsley, if using.

Makes 4 servings

Source: Bureau of Markets/Farmers' Markets

Italian Basil Tomato Salad

4 medium tomatoes
2 tablespoons vegetable oil
3 tablespoons red wine vinegar
5 to 6 chopped fresh basil leaves
Salt and black pepper

Cut the tomatoes into thin wedges or slices and spread them out over a wide, shallow bowl. In a small bowl, whisk together the remaining ingredients with salt and pepper to taste and pour over the tomatoes. Baste the tomatoes with the dressing by tilting the dish and spooning it over the tomatoes repeatedly. Marinate for 20 to 30 minutes before serving.

Makes 4 servings

Source: Bureau of Markets/Farmers' Markets

Bulgur Wheat with Vegetables

2 tablespoons unsalted butter
1 cup uncooked bulgur wheat
1 medium onion, chopped
1 cup thinly sliced celery
½ cup diced red bell pepper
¾ teaspoon ground cumin
1 teaspoon chili powder
2¼ cups low-sodium beef broth or water
Salt and black pepper

In a large skillet, melt the butter over medium heat. Add the bulgur and onion and cook until the onion is softened and the bulgur is golden, about 5 minutes. Stir in the celery, red pepper, cumin, and chili powder and cook for 2 minutes. Stir in the beef broth and bring to a boil. Reduce the heat and simmer for about 20 minutes, or until all the liquid is absorbed. Season with salt and black pepper to taste.

Makes 6 servings

Recipe courtesy of the Wheat Foods Council

Marinated Brussels Sprouts

1 pound Brussels sprouts
½ cup oil
¼ cup vinegar
½ teaspoon Dijon mustard
½ teaspoon garlic powder
½ teaspoon black pepper

Bring a large pot of water to a boil. Add the Brussels sprouts and cook until just barely tender, about 6 to 8 minutes. Drain and place in a large bowl.

In a medium bowl, whisk together the remaining ingredients. Pour over the cooked Brussels sprouts while they are still warm. Cover and refrigerate for at least 4 hours before serving.

Makes 4 to 6 servings

Source: Bureau of Markets/Farmers' Markets

BRAIN POWER ENTRÉES

Fast and Fit Clam Chowder

1 tablespoon unsalted butter or margarine

1 cup chopped leeks or onions

1 cup diced red or green bell peppers or a combination

Two 6½-ounce cans chopped clams in clam juice

2 pounds (about 6 medium) potatoes, cut into ½-inch cubes

One 14½-ounce can low-sodium chicken broth

2 teaspoons dried thyme

1 cup lowfat milk

One 10-ounce package frozen corn kernels, thawed and drained

⅛ teaspoon cayenne pepper

Salt and black pepper

Cheddar cheese, to serve (optional)

Chopped fresh parsley, to serve (optional)

Crumbled cooked bacon, to serve (optional)

Place the butter in a 2½- to 3-quart microwave-safe bowl. Microwave on high for 1 minute. Add the leeks and bell peppers and microwave on high for 3 minutes. Drain the juice from the clams into the microwaved vegetables, reserving the clams. Stir in the potatoes, broth, and thyme. Cover with plastic wrap, venting one corner. Microwave on high for 20 minutes. Using a slotted spoon, remove 4 cups of the cooked potatoes; set aside. Pour the contents of the bowl into a blender. Add the milk and, holding the lid down tightly, blend until smooth. Return the mixture to the bowl. Stir in the reserved clams and potatoes, the corn, and cayenne. Season with salt and pepper to taste. Microwave on high for 3 minutes, or until heated through. If you like, pass around bowls of shredded cheddar cheese, chopped parsley, and/or crumbled cooked bacon to stir into the soup.

Makes 4 servings

Recipe courtesy of the Northern Plains Potato Growers Association

Crab Cakes

2 slices stale bread, crusts removed

Small amount of milk (about ¼ cup)

1 tablespoon mayonnaise

1 tablespoon Worcestershire sauce

1 tablespoon parsley flakes

1 tablespoon baking powder

1 teaspoon Old Bay seasoning

¼ teaspoon salt

1 large egg, beaten

1 pound fresh lump crabmeat

¼ cup olive oil

Break the bread into small pieces and place in a large bowl. Moisten the bread with the milk. Add the remaining ingredients and mix together well. Shape into patties. Fry in olive oil on both sides about 6 to 8 minutes each side, or until golden brown. Serve with cocktail sauce or tartar sauce.

Makes 4 servings

Recipe courtesy of the Restaurant Association of Maryland

Apricot-Glazed Pork Kabobs

One 10-ounce jar apricot preserves
4 tablespoons orange liqueur or orange juice
2 tablespoons unsalted butter
1 pound boneless pork loin, cut into 1-inch cubes

Preheat the barbecue or grill.

In a small saucepan, combine the apricot preserves, orange liqueur, and butter. Place over medium heat and bring to a simmer. Simmer until the butter is melted. Cool. (Alternatively, combine the ingredients in a 2-cup glass measure and microwave on high for 1 minute.) Place the pork cubes in a heavy-duty zip-top bag, along with ¾ cup of the apricot mixture. Turn the mixture to coat and marinate for 30 minutes. Thread the pork cubes onto skewers (if using bamboo skewers, soak them in water for 30 minutes before using to prevent burning).

Grill for 10 to 12 minutes, turning occasionally and basting often with the marinade. In a medium saucepan over medium heat, warm the remaining apricot mixture to boiling and serve alongside the kabobs, if you like.

Makes 4 servings

Recipe courtesy of the Minnesota Pork Board

Baked Pork Chops

6 lean, center-cut, ½-inch-thick pork chops
1 medium onion, thinly sliced
½ cup chopped green bell pepper
½ cup chopped red bell pepper
¼ teaspoon salt
⅛ teaspoon black pepper
Chopped fresh parsley, to garnish

Preheat the oven to 375°F.

Trim the fat from the pork chops and place the chops in a 13×9-inch baking pan. Spread the onion and bell peppers on top of the pork chops. Sprinkle with salt and pepper. Refrigerate for 1 hour.

Cover the pan with foil and bake for 30 minutes. Uncover the pan, turn the pork chops, and bake for an additional 15 minutes, or until no pink remains. Garnish with the parsley and serve.

Makes 6 servings

Source: Food Stamp Nutrition Connection

Spaghetti Squash–Stuffed Peppers

Nonstick cooking spray
¼ cup low-sodium chicken broth
1 cup chopped zucchini or yellow crookneck squash
½ cup chopped shiitake or button mushrooms
¼ cup thinly sliced green onions
1 tablespoon chopped fresh basil or 1 teaspoon crumbled dried basil
1 tablespoon chopped fresh thyme or 1 teaspoon crumbled
   dried thyme

1 clove garlic, minced
¼ teaspoon black pepper
1½ cups cooked spaghetti squash (fluffed into strands)
4 bell peppers (any color)
¼ cup shredded nonfat or lowfat Swiss or cheddar cheese

Preheat the oven to 375°F. Coat a small baking dish with cooking spray.

In a large skillet over medium heat, heat the chicken broth to a simmer. Add the zucchini, mushrooms, green onions, basil, thyme, garlic, and pepper. Simmer, uncovered, stirring occasionally, for 4 minutes, or until the vegetables are tender. Remove from the heat and stir in the spaghetti squash. Slice the tops off the bell peppers and discard the seeds and membranes. Spoon the filling into the bell peppers and sprinkle on the shredded cheese. Replace the tops. Place in the baking dish, cover with foil, and bake for 30 to 35 minutes, or until heated through.

Makes 4 servings

Recipe courtesy of the Georgia Fruit and Vegetable Growers Association

ENERGIZING DESSERTS

Chocolate Pudding Surprise

8 ounces cooked sweet potatoes, chopped (about 1 cup)
4 ounces reduced-fat cream cheese (not nonfat)
½ cup lowfat vanilla yogurt
¼ cup brown sugar
½ cup chocolate syrup

Whipped topping, to serve (optional)
Crumbled chocolate cream-filled sandwich cookies, to serve
(optional)

Place the sweet potatoes in a food processor and purée. Add
the remaining ingredients and process until smooth and creamy.
Spoon into dessert dishes. Refrigerate before serving. If desired,
garnish with whipped topping and crumbled chocolate cream-
filled sandwich cookies.

Makes 4 servings

Recipe courtesy of the North Carolina Sweet Potato Commission

Fruit Yogurt Pudding

¾ cup sliced fresh seasonal fruit (such as strawberries, raspberries, blueberries, apples, peaches, or pears)
2 teaspoons fresh lemon juice
½ cup lowfat plain or vanilla yogurt
½ cup (4 ounces) lowfat cottage cheese
2 teaspoons honey
½ teaspoon vanilla extract

Line the bottom of a serving bowl with the fruit. Drizzle the
lemon juice over the fruit. In a medium bowl, whip together
the yogurt, cottage cheese, honey, and vanilla. Cover the fruit
with the yogurt mixture and refrigerate for several hours before
serving.

Makes 2 servings

Source: Bureau of Markets/Farmers' Markets

Novi's Prune Fudge Pie

½ cup cognac

1 pound moist or ½ pound dried prunes

3 ounces semisweet chocolate

2 sticks unsalted butter or margarine

2 cups rice syrup (see note below)

6 large eggs

¼ teaspoon salt

¼ teaspoon vanilla extract

2 unbaked 9-inch pie shells

Whipped cream, to serve

Preheat the oven to 350°F.

Place the cognac in a medium bowl. Mince the prunes, then soak them in the cognac. If moist prunes are used, soak for 1 hour; if the prunes are dried, soak them overnight.

In a medium saucepan over medium-low heat, melt the chocolate and butter together. Pour into a large bowl. Add the rice syrup, eggs, salt, vanilla, and prunes with the cognac and mix well. Pour into the pie shells and bake for 60 minutes, or until a knife inserted near the center comes out clean.

Cool to room temperature, then refrigerate. Serve chilled with whipped cream.

Makes 16 servings

Note: Rice syrup is available in health food stores. Alternatively, you can substitute 2 cups of sugar and reduce the amount of eggs to 4.

Recipe courtesy of Sunsweet Growers Inc.

Orange Banana Frosty

1 banana, peeled, cut into chunks, and frozen
½ cup lowfat plain yogurt
½ cup orange juice

Put all the ingredients in a blender and blend. Add more liquid if you'd like a thinner consistency. Pour into glasses and serve immediately.

Makes 2 servings

Source: Food Stamp Nutrition Connection

Famous Banana Dessert

2 cups skim or lowfat milk
One 3½-ounce box banana or vanilla instant pudding mix
1 cup nonfat yogurt or nondairy whipped topping
2 bananas, sliced, or other fruit slices

In a medium bowl, combine the milk and pudding mix. Beat with wooden spoon, wire whisk, or electric mixer on the lowest speed for 2 minutes. Gently mix the yogurt with the pudding mixture. Cover and refrigerate for 30 minutes. Layer fruit slices in the bottom of 8 dessert cups. Pour the pudding mixture over the sliced fruit. Refrigerate until ready to serve, at least 5 minutes, though it's best if refrigerated a bit longer.

Makes 8 servings

Source: Food Stamp Nutrition Connection

THREE

❋

Cooking Up Answers to Addictions

Food is medicine. It's a fact that proper diet and nutrition are essential components to treating countless diseases and conditions, including heart disease, diabetes, high blood pressure, and arthritis, to name just a few. But did you know that food can be used to treat addictions, too? This makes perfect sense, if you consider that people who are addicted to drugs and alcohol are among the most undernourished patients in health care. Nutrition should be an integral part of the healing process—and in effective recovery programs, it is. Food is an unsung hero when it comes to addictions.

Eating healthy foods won't necessarily break the hold of an addiction, but it will help rebuild a body nutritionally depleted by substance abuse. What you may not realize is that alcohol, nicotine, and illicit drugs destroy nutrients, prevent their absorption, and flush them from the body. Cocaine and heroin addiction, in particular, reduce the intake of nutritious foods and cause serious malnutrition, whereas marijuana creates an abnormally large appetite for sweets and snacks, leading to unhealthy weight gain. In large amounts, alcohol flushes many nutrients from the body, including thiamine, vitamin B_6, and calcium. Smoking robs the body of vital, disease-fighting antioxidants, including vitamin C. These deficiencies can remain, even if you stop using a substance, giving rise to imbalances that lead to serious illnesses such as cancer, kidney and liver diseases, and heart disease, and thus creating a greater crisis to manage. If you or a loved one is in a recovery program, you'll want to use nutrition as one of the tools to get better, and the foods and recipes in this chapter can help.

A case that comes to mind is Jack, an extremely smart man who had earned two Ph.D.s in his lifetime. After discovering that both of his ex-wives had cheated on him, he began drinking heavily, and his drinking, usually done alone, progressed to alcoholism. We find malnutrition in every addict we see, and Jack was no different. Alcoholics tend to eat poorly and may become depleted of many nutrients, often with disastrous results if not treated. Jack had developed an alcohol-related disease called chronic alcoholic myopathy, a condition in which alcohol begins to destroy muscle tissue, and weakness gradually develops over weeks or months. The nerves of the extremities may also begin to break down, a condition known as alcoholic peripheral neuropathy, which can add to the person's difficulty in moving. Fortunately, Jack entered rehabilitation just in the nick of time. Chronic alcoholic myopathy can be treated successfully by correcting nutritional deficiencies and maintaining a diet adequate in protein and carbohydrates. Jack was put on a special diet to accomplish this, in addition to undergoing a behavioral program to help him overcome his alcohol addiction. It was a long road to recovery, but Jack made it. Most patients recover fully from acute alcoholic myopathy, and Jack was no exception. Today he remains alcohol-free.

Chronic drug abuse can mangle brain function so profoundly that the addict's judgment is altered, making him or her more prone to poor choices, including nutritional choices. In the addiction program I (Frank) supervised in New Mexico years ago, it was critical for patients to undergo dietary therapy so that they could regain their common sense abilities as soon as possible and start selecting foods that could assist the body in healing. Dietary therapy remains one of the most important elements of the rehabilitation process, since it has the power to correct nutritional shortfalls, improve a person's brain function, and support physical healing.

If you're being treated for or recovering from an addiction, nutrition can help usher in a whole new way of life for a more successful recovery. Here are some important points to keep in mind.

Follow a Diet High in Protein

Inside your body a marvelous process of self-repair takes place, day in and day out, and it all has to do with protein, the nutrient responsible for building and maintaining body tissues. You'll want to make sure that protein comprises about 20 to 25 percent of your total daily calories. If you don't like counting or weighing foods, have the protein equivalent of three decks of cards each day, or have a few ounces of protein at each meal. Good choices include lean meat, poultry, fish, lowfat dairy products, and vegetable protein such as legumes or tofu.

Eat Foods Rich in Vitamin A

Vitamin A is also involved in the growth and repair of tissues; in addition, it increases resistance to infection. Addictions lower your immune defenses, so you'll want to ramp up this important vitamin. It is found primarily in animal sources such as fish, liver, milk, butter, and eggs. Orange-hued foods such as carrots and sweet potatoes contain beta-carotene, which converts to vitamin A in the body, so pile these vegetables on your plate as often as you can.

Include Foods High in B Vitamins

In this family of nutrients, there are eight major B-complex vitamins—thiamin, riboflavin, niacin, vitamin B_{12}, folic acid, pyridoxine, pantothenic acid, and biotin—that work in accord to ensure proper digestion, muscle contraction, and energy production. Whole grains, vegetables, lean meats, and legumes are good sources. This family of vitamins is essential for helping to restore liver function, a concern with alcohol addiction.

Enjoy Generous Amounts of Foods Rich in Vitamin C

Take a cue from the many doctors who treat addictions by prescribing high doses of vitamin C for detoxification, and include vitamin C–rich foods in your diet. The best sources of vitamin C in the diet are citrus fruits. Other foods, such as green and red bell peppers, collard greens, broccoli, Brussels sprouts, cabbage, spinach, potatoes, cantaloupe, and strawberries are also excel-

lent sources. Another excellent source of vitamin C is the artichoke, also widely valued for its healing effect on the liver.
Vitamin C, incidentally, is drastically depleted in smokers, so
this strategy is all the more important if you smoke.

Go Raw

A natural foods diet that includes raw fruits and vegetables is
often recommended as nutritional support in treating addictions and restoring health. Fresh fruits and vegetables, such as
apples, pears, pineapples, salad greens, and dark-green leafy vegetables such as broccoli, kale, cabbage, and spinach are full of
nutrients that help reduce the risks of heart disease and certain
cancers. If you're not a big fan of vegetables, try drinking them
in the form of a fresh juice. Drinking fresh vegetable juices is
one of the best ways to infuse your body with a healthful concentration of nutrients and will go a long way toward nutritional healing.

Basically, an all-around nutritious diet with a wide variety of
foods is key to overturning the damage caused by an addiction.
The recipes in this chapter incorporate a number of healthy,
nutrition-packed foods that can serve as the basis for such a diet.

SMART TIPS ⊛ **KICKING ADDICTIONS**

- Acknowledge your problem. Go to a professional and be evalu-
  ated as to whether you have an addiction, a compulsion, or other
  problems.

continued

- Get a plan, find help, and start moving immediately into the steps of recovery. Your plan may involve supportive psychotherapy, medical care, and family support to help you return to productive living.

- Consider joining a self-help group that includes people with similar addictive problems. A psychologist can help you identify which type of group might be best for you.

- Enroll in yoga classes. Clinical research with yoga as a complementary treatment for all sorts of addictions has been impressive.

- If you relapse, keep trying. Never give up.

STARTERS AND OTHER DELIGHTS

Orange Cider

3 cups orange juice
1 cup apple juice
One 2-inch cinnamon stick
¼ teaspoon whole cloves
Orange slices, to serve (optional)

In a medium saucepan, combine the orange juice, apple juice, cinnamon, and cloves. Bring to a boil over medium-high heat. Reduce the heat, cover, and simmer for 10 minutes. Remove the cinnamon stick and cloves. Pour into mugs and serve warm. If you like, float some orange slices on top.

Makes 4 servings

Recipe courtesy of the Florida Department of Citrus Headquarters

Paradise Island

½ cup orange juice
½ cup grapefruit juice
½ cup frozen strawberries

In a blender, combine the orange juice, grapefruit juice, and frozen strawberries. Blend until smooth. Pour into glasses and serve immediately.

Makes 2 servings

Recipe courtesy of the Florida Department of Citrus Headquarters

Super-Juice Tonic

3 carrots (include the tops if you have them)
½ cucumber
½ beet with greens
5 asparagus spears

Run all the ingredients through an electric juicer, cutting the vegetables to fit if necessary. Pour into a glass and serve immediately.

Makes 1 large serving

Recipe courtesy of Maggie Greenwood-Robinson

Artichokes with Garlic Dip

1 cup lowfat plain yogurt
1 tablespoon chopped fresh parsley
1 tablespoon chopped fresh chives

2 teaspoons chili sauce
2 cloves garlic, minced
⅛ teaspoon black pepper
4 medium cooked artichokes

Combine all the ingredients except the artichokes in a blender and blend well. Refrigerate until serving. Serve the artichokes with the dip.

Makes 4 servings

Source: Centers for Disease Control

Shiitake, Artichoke, and Fontina Fondue

4 cups (about 1 pound) shredded fontina cheese
1 tablespoon cornstarch
2 tablespoons unsalted butter
1½ cups (about 6 ounces) finely chopped shiitake mushrooms
2 tablespoons finely chopped shallots
1 cup finely chopped canned artichoke hearts
½ cup dry white wine
½ cup low-sodium chicken broth
¼ cup fresh lemon juice
1 tablespoon fresh thyme leaves or 1 teaspoon dried thyme
½ teaspoon salt
Freshly ground black pepper
For Dipping: Boiled peeled shrimp, steamed small red-skinned
    potatoes, onion and herb focaccia cut into bite-size pieces

In a medium bowl, toss the cheese with the cornstarch. In a medium heavy-bottomed saucepan, heat the butter over medium heat. Add the mushrooms and shallots and sauté for 3 to 4 minutes, until softened. Add the artichoke hearts and cook for another 3 minutes. Stir in the wine, chicken broth, and lemon juice and heat until just barely simmering. Add the cheese, a handful at a time, stirring until the cheese is melted before adding more. When all the cheese has been added, stir in the thyme, salt, and pepper.

Transfer the fondue to an enamel or ceramic fondue pot and keep warm over a fondue burner. Serve immediately with your choice of dippers.

Makes 12 servings

Recipe Courtesy of the Midwest Dairy Association

SMART SIDE DISHES

Quick Sweet-Sour Cabbage

1 tablespoon brown sugar
1 tablespoon apple cider vinegar
1 tablespoon cornstarch
⅛ teaspoon salt
1 cup orange juice
5 cups packaged shredded cabbage and carrot mix
One 2-ounce jar diced pimientos, drained

In a small bowl, combine the brown sugar, vinegar, cornstarch, and salt; set aside. In a large saucepan over medium-high heat, bring the orange juice to a boil. Add the cabbage and pimientos. Return to a boil and add the sugar-vinegar mixture. Cook, stirring, until thickened and bubbly.

Makes 4 servings

Recipe courtesy of the Florida Department of Citrus Headquarters

Orange-Zucchini Pasta

1 cup dried cavatelli, medium shell macaroni, rotini,
*   or radiatore pasta*
1 large onion, cut into thin wedges
One 14½-ounce can chunky pasta-style tomatoes
¾ cup orange juice
1 large zucchini, halved lengthwise and cut into ¼-inch-thick
*   slices*
Dash of black pepper

Cook the pasta according to package directions, adding the onion during the last 5 minutes of cooking. Drain. Set aside and keep warm.

Meanwhile, in a large skillet over medium-high heat, combine the tomatoes and orange juice and bring to a boil. Boil, uncovered, for 5 to 6 minutes, until slightly thickened. Add the zucchini and pepper to the skillet and return to a boil. Reduce the heat and simmer, uncovered, for about 3 minutes, or until the zucchini is crisp-tender. Stir in the pasta and onion and heat through.

Makes 4 servings

Recipe courtesy of the Florida Department of Citrus Headquarters

Artichoke and Roasted Red Pepper Salad
with Roasted Pepper Dressing

SALAD

8 medium cooked artichokes

3 red bell peppers

8 lettuce leaves, to serve

½ cup sliced red onion

½ cup sliced black olives

DRESSING

Reserved roasted bell pepper from the salad preparation

⅓ cup balsamic vinegar

¼ cup olive oil

2 cloves garlic, minced

1 tablespoon chopped fresh basil or 1 teaspoon crushed
dried basil

1 teaspoon chopped fresh rosemary or ½ teaspoon crushed dried
rosemary

To make the salad, preheat the broiler to high. Halve the artichokes lengthwise and scoop out the center petals and fuzzy centers. Remove the outer leaves and reserve to garnish the salad, or save for another time. Trim out the hearts and slice thinly. Cover and set aside.

Place the bell peppers under the broiler and broil until charred on all sides, turning frequently with tongs. Remove from the oven and place in a paper bag for 15 minutes to steam the skins. Remove the stems, seeds, and ribs. Strip off skins and thinly slice the bell peppers. Reserve a quarter of the bell pepper strips to prepare dressing. To assemble the salads, arrange the lettuce leaves over 8 salad plates. Arrange the sliced artichoke hearts, remaining bell pepper strips, and red onion and olive slices over the lettuce. Garnish with a couple of cooked artichoke leaves if you like.

For the dressing, place the reserved bell pepper strips, vinegar, olive oil, garlic, basil, and rosemary in a blender or food processor. Blend until nearly smooth. Spoon the dressing over the salads.

Makes 8 servings

Source: Centers for Disease Control

Sweet Potato Salad

2½ pounds sweet potatoes
2 medium unpeeled tart green apples, cored and cut into
    ½-inch dice
1 small fresh pineapple, peeled and cut into ½-inch chunks,
    or one 20-ounce can pineapple chunks
½ cup golden raisins
¾ cup mayonnaise
¾ cup plain yogurt
1½ tablespoons curry powder
½ teaspoon salt

Place the sweet potatoes in a large saucepan with salted water to cover. Bring to a boil, then reduce the heat and simmer, covered, until just tender, 15 to 20 minutes. Drain the sweet potatoes well and peel while still warm.

Cool completely, then cut into ¾-inch chunks and place in a large bowl. Add the apples, pineapple, and raisins; set aside. In a small bowl, whisk together the mayonnaise, yogurt, curry powder, and salt. Add to the potato mixture and toss gently until well combined. Chill for at least 1 hour before serving.

Makes 6 to 8 servings

Source: Centers for Disease Control

Spicy Apple-Filled Squash

1 acorn squash (about 1 pound)
1 Golden Delicious apple, peeled, cored, and sliced
2 teaspoons reduced-fat margarine, melted
2 teaspoons brown sugar
⅛ teaspoon ground cinnamon
⅛ teaspoon ground nutmeg
Dash of ground cloves

Preheat the oven to 350°F. Grease a 1-quart baking dish.

Halve the squash, remove the seeds, and cut into quarters. Place the quarters, skin side up, in the baking dish, cover with foil, and bake for 30 minutes.

Meanwhile, in a medium bowl, combine the apple, margarine, brown sugar, cinnamon, nutmeg, and cloves. Remove the squash from the oven and turn so the flesh is facing up. Top with apple mixture, cover again, and bake for 30 minutes longer, or until the apples are tender.

For a quick microwave version, arrange the squash quarters, cut side up, in a microwave-safe baking dish. Microwave on high for 6 to 7 minutes, until softened, rotating the squash halfway through cooking time. Top the squash with the apple mixture, cover with vented plastic wrap, and microwave on high for 4 to 5 minutes, until the apples are tender.

Makes 2 servings

Source: Centers for Disease Control

BRAIN POWER ENTRÉES

Broiled Fish with Citrus-Grape Sauce

Nonstick cooking spray
2 pounds fresh or frozen grouper, halibut, or shark steak, about
   ¾ inch thick
1 teaspoon lemon-pepper seasoning
¼ cup thinly sliced green onions
½ teaspoon grated orange zest
1¼ cups orange juice
1 tablespoon cornstarch
¼ teaspoon salt
3 oranges, peeled, sectioned, and seeded
1 cup seedless green grapes, halved
2 tablespoons dry sherry (optional)

Preheat the broiler.

Spray the rack of a broiler pan with cooking spray. Sprinkle both sides of the fish with lemon-pepper seasoning. Place the fish on the rack of the broiler pan. Broil 4 inches from the heat for 4 minutes. Turn the fish and broil 3 to 5 minutes more, until the fish flakes when tested with a fork.

Meanwhile, spray a medium saucepan with nonstick coating. Add the green onions and place over medium heat. Sauté the green onions until softened, about 5 minutes.

In a small bowl, combine the orange zest, orange juice, corn-starch, and salt. Add to the green onions and cook, stirring, until the mixture is thickened and bubbly, then cook, stirring for 2 minutes more. Add the orange sections, grapes, and sherry, if using, and heat through. Remove the fish to a serving platter and spoon the sauce over the fish.

Makes 4 servings

Recipe courtesy of the Florida Department of Citrus Headquarters

Grilled Halibut

½ cup grapefruit juice
¼ cup olive oil
2 teaspoons chopped fresh marjoram
½ teaspoon salt
⅛ teaspoon black pepper
Four 8-ounce halibut steaks
Grapefruit sections, to serve

In a shallow glass dish, mix together the grapefruit juice, oil, marjoram, salt, and pepper. Add the fish, turning once to coat both sides, then cover the dish and refrigerate for 1 to 2 hours, turning once or twice.

Set up the barbecue and place the grill 4 to 6 inches above the coals, or preheat a gas grill. Grill the fish for 10 to 12 minutes, turning once and brushing twice with remaining marinade, until the steaks are barely opaque in the thickest part. Arrange on a platter and scatter grapefruit sections around the steaks.

Makes 4 servings

Recipe courtesy of the Florida Department of Citrus Headquarters

Vegetarian Paella

1½ *tablespoons olive oil*
1 *large onion, chopped*
½ *teaspoon paprika*
1½ *cups uncooked long-grain brown rice*
3¾ *cups low-sodium vegetable broth*
¾ *cup dry white wine*
One 14-ounce can chopped tomatoes with juice
1 *tablespoon tomato paste*
½ *teaspoon dried tarragon*
1 *teaspoon dried basil*
1 *teaspoon dried oregano*
1 *red bell pepper, roughly chopped*
1 *green bell pepper, roughly chopped*
3 *ribs celery, finely chopped*
3 *cups sliced button mushrooms*
½ *cup snow peas*
⅔ *cup frozen peas*
⅓ *cup cashew pieces*
Salt and black pepper

In a large, deep skillet, heat the oil over medium heat. Add the onions and sauté until softened, about 5 minutes. Add the paprika and rice and cook for 4 to 5 minutes, stirring occasionally, until the rice is transparent. Add the broth, wine, tomatoes, tomato paste, tarragon, basil, and oregano, bring to a simmer, and simmer for 10 to 15 minutes. Add the bell peppers, celery, mushrooms, and snow peas and cook for another 30 minutes, or until the rice is cooked. Add the peas and cashews and the salt and pepper to taste. Cook to heat through, then place on a large heated serving dish to serve.

Makes 4 servings

Source: Centers for Disease Control

One-Pot Lentil Stew

1 cup dried lentils, rinsed
½ cup uncooked brown rice
3 cups sliced carrots
1 pound Swiss chard, chopped
1 pound kale, chopped
3 cups water
1 regular-size packet onion soup mix
1 teaspoon dried basil
1 tablespoon olive oil

Place all the ingredients in a large pot. Place over medium-high heat and bring to a boil. Reduce the heat and cook until the mixture has a stewlike consistency.

Makes 6 servings

Source: Centers for Disease Control

Baked Tofu

One 16-ounce package firm or extra-firm tofu, drained
2 tablespoons soy sauce
1 clove garlic, minced, or ¼ teaspoon garlic powder
1 teaspoon minced fresh ginger (optional)
1 teaspoon vegetable oil

Preheat the oven to 350°F. Line a rimmed baking sheet with foil. Wrap the tofu in paper towel to absorb excess water. Let set for about 5 minutes.

While the tofu is draining, in a small bowl, combine the soy sauce, garlic, ginger, and oil. Cut the tofu into ½-inch-thick slices and place the tofu slices on the foil-lined baking sheet. Pour the soy sauce mixture over the tofu. Using a spatula or pancake turner, gently turn the slices over to coat both sides with the sauce.

Place in the oven and bake for 15 minutes, then turn the slices over and bake for another 15 minutes, or until the tofu is light golden brown and firm. Serve hot in place of a meat entrée or cut into cubes and add to a stir-fry, fried rice, soup, or salad.

Makes 4 servings

Source: Food Stamp Nutrition Connection

ENERGIZING DESSERTS

Orange-Berry Tart

Pastry for Single-Crust Pie (recipe follows)

FILLING

One 8-ounce package reduced-fat cream cheese, softened
¼ cup sugar
1 tablespoon orange juice
1 teaspoon grated orange zest

ORANGE GLAZE

⅔ cup orange juice
1 tablespoon sugar
2 teaspoons cornstarch
2 oranges, peeled, sectioned, and seeded
1 pint strawberries, hulled and halved
Thin strips of orange peel (optional)
Thin strips of lime peel (optional)

Preheat the oven to 450°F.

Prepare the pastry for a Single-Crust Pie. On a lightly floured surface, flatten the ball of dough with your hands. Roll the dough from the center out, forming a circle about 13 inches in diameter. Ease the pastry into an 11-inch tart pan with a removable bottom, being careful not to stretch the pastry. Trim even with the edge of the pan. Prick bottom and sides of the pastry generously with the tines of a fork. Bake for 10 to 12 minutes, until golden. Cool the pastry completely on a wire rack.

For the filling, in a medium bowl, combine the cream cheese, sugar, and orange juice. Beat with an electric mixer on high speed until light and fluffy. Stir in the orange zest. Spread the filling over the baked tart shell.

For the orange glaze, in a small saucepan, combine the orange juice, sugar, and cornstarch. Cook, stirring, over medium heat until the mixture is thickened and bubbly, then cook, stirring, for 2 minutes more. Remove from the heat and cool completely.

Arrange the orange sections, followed by the strawberry halves on top of the cream cheese filling. Spread the orange glaze over all. Sprinkle with the orange peel and lime peel, if using. Cover and refrigerate for up to 6 hours. Remove sides of pan from the tart and place the tart on serving plate.

Makes 10 servings

Pastry for Single-Crust Pie

1¼ cups all-purpose flour
¼ teaspoon salt
¼ cup shortening
4 to 5 tablespoons cold water

In a medium bowl stir together the flour and salt. Cut in the shortening until the mixture resembles fine crumbs. Sprinkle 1 tablespoon of the water at a time over the mixture and gently toss with a fork. Push the moistened dough to the side of the bowl and repeat until all the dough is moistened. Form the dough into a ball.

Recipe courtesy of the Florida Department of Citrus Headquarters

Raw Fudge

2 cups cashews, soaked overnight
1 cup pitted dates
1 cup dried unsweetened cranberries
2 heaping tablespoons cocoa powder
½ cup pomegranate juice
½ cup water
1 cup flax seed meal
1 cup chopped walnuts

Drain the cashews and place in a blender or food processor with the dates, cranberries, cocoa powder, pomegranate juice, and water. Blend until the mixture forms a thick paste. Place in a bowl and stir in the flax seed meal and water. Refrigerate for 2 hours. Cut into squares and store in the freezer.

Makes 12 servings

Recipe Courtesy of Maggie Greenwood-Robinson

Savory Fresh Apricot Bites

4 ounces fat-free cream cheese, softened
12 fresh apricots, halved
¼ cup finely chopped pistachios

In a small bowl, stir the cream cheese until smooth; pipe through a pastry bag or spoon into the apricot halves. Sprinkle the tops with pistachios.

Makes 6 servings

Source: Centers for Disease Control

Maggie's Apple Crisp

Nonstick cooking spray
2 tablespoons rolled oats
2 tablespoons toasted wheat germ
¼ cup all-purpose wheat flour
¼ cup firmly packed light brown sugar
½ teaspoon ground cinnamon
¼ teaspoon ground nutmeg
1½ tablespoons unsalted butter, softened
4 medium apples
2 cups nonfat vanilla frozen yogurt

Preheat the oven to 375°F. Coat an 8×8-inch baking pan with cooking spray.

In a medium bowl, thoroughly combine the oats, wheat germ, flour, brown sugar, cinnamon, and nutmeg.

Peel, core, and thinly slice the apples. Spread the apple slices evenly over the surface of the baking pan. Sprinkle the oat-flour mixture over the apples. Dot the mixture with bits of butter. Place in the oven and bake for 30 minutes, or until the apples are tender and the topping is golden brown.

Serve warm, topping each serving with ¼ cup frozen yogurt.

Makes 8 servings

Recipe courtesy Maggie of Greenwood-Robinson

Instant Chocolate Mousse

1 small box (3½-ounces) instant chocolate pudding mix
1¼ cups soymilk, chilled
One 10½-ounce package silken tofu

Place the chocolate pudding mix and soymilk in a medium bowl. Using an electric mixer, beat on medium speed for about 15 seconds, or until the mixture is very smooth. Add the tofu and blend again until very smooth, scraping the sides of the bowl if needed to make sure it's all mixed in. Pour the mixture into 4 small serving dishes, cover with plastic, and refrigerate for at least 2 hours before serving.

Makes 4 servings

Source: Food Stamp Nutrition Connection

FOUR

※

Dish Up More Concentration

Do your thoughts scatter like marbles much of the time? Are you easily distracted? Is getting organized or setting priorities tough for you? Can you remember to add the correct numbers together? Do you finish your tasks, or are they half-finished messes?

If so, you may have an attention problem that, well, needs attention. You can start by making some adjustments to your diet. A healthy diet, including a good breakfast, is important for both children and adults to maximize concentration, learning capacity, and alertness.

At least 90 percent of children and adults who come to our clinic in Texas for problems with attention and concentration have very poor diets, loaded with sugar and unhealthy trans fats, which are found in many snack foods and processed foods. These ingredients can have a disastrous impact on concentration and must be eliminated in order for the brain to process with speed and focus. As evidence, schools across the country that have started serving healthier foods and eliminating fast foods from their cafeterias have seen a 10 to 20 percent improvement in academic performance.

There is a close connection between food and attention span. If you're interested in staying mentally alert and keeping your kids focused, too, try the following diet suggestions.

Go Higher Protein at Breakfast

To get clients on the path to better brain health, we ask that each person who comes to the clinic for attention problems eat a breakfast with at least 50 percent protein, including foods such as cheese, Canadian bacon, lowfat ham, eggs (boiled), or peanut butter. A higher-protein diet shifts the brain into focus mode. Protein-rich foods supply tyrosine, which has been linked to increased alertness. Many proteins, such as lean red meat, are rich in iron, too. When iron is in short supply, attention and learning are impeded.

Recently we saw a miracle take place in a sweet, charming boy named Gus. His parents brought him to us because he was sleepy throughout much of his school day. Every time he'd sit down for a task, he'd quickly dose off. After questioning his parents about his diet, we discovered that he ate doughnuts for breakfast and candy bars at lunch. We recommended that he start the day with a high-protein breakfast. Bingo. The very first day Gus tried this, he was alert in school and in a much more upbeat mood. His grades soon got better, and he felt energetic enough to get involved in sports. A simple adjustment in his diet made all the difference in the world.

There are mounds of research proving how important breakfast is, especially to kids. We can sum it up like this: Skip breakfast and mental performance deteriorates. Eat a healthy breakfast and expect needle-sharp thinking throughout the day. That goes not only for kids, but for adults, too.

Reduce Sugars

Simple sugars are processed rapidly by the body, causing highs and lows in energy. Low blood sugar in particular has a depressant effect on the body and can make you feel blue.

Simple sugars include white sugar, brown sugar, honey, corn syrup, and cane sugar. They are fine for sweetening foods, but they should be used sparingly. Starches such as pasta and potatoes are complex sugars that are broken down more slowly, creating a more stable supply of glucose and supplying a more appropriate level of mental stimulation. Fruits contain carbohydrates and fiber and are an excellent source of minerals and vitamins, which have many positive attributes for the body. Fruits contain natural sugars, which are preferable to the simple sugars listed above.

Parents often ask whether sugar makes kids hyperactive. Keep in mind that all children are highly energetic at times. But that doesn't make them hyperactive. The term *hyperactivity*, or attention deficit/hyperactivity disorder (ADHD), is used by psychologists to define a specific type of behavioral problem. It includes inattention, impulsive behavior, and significantly increased activity.

Research on sugar and hyperactivity is mixed and can be confusing. We recommend staying on the safe side. Restrict sugar in your child's diet to an occasional treat, and replace the sugar with fresh fruit.

What the research does clearly suggest is that healthy dietary habits are the best way to ensure optimal mental and behavioral performance at all times. Your goal for you and your family should be to emphasize foods that provide a broad array of vitamins and minerals, and to eat fresh fruits, vegetables, whole grains, and cereals regularly.

Be Sure to Get Enough B$_6$

One vitamin that is particularly important, especially in kids with attention problems, is vitamin B$_6$, as it enhances the effects of other vitamins and minerals. It also helps combat an assortment of diseases. It is one of the most studied vitamins, and lack of it is believed to contribute to a wide range of health and mental problems, including seizures, autism, depression, headaches, poor memory, agitated behavior, anxiety, and sleep difficulties.

Children with ADD often have low levels of vitamin B$_6$. When those levels are raised, their concentration often improves. Foods high in vitamin B$_6$ are among the many featured in this cookbook: bananas, chickpeas, potatoes, chicken, oatmeal, pork loin, peanut butter, and walnuts.

Vitamins and minerals are not a cure for attention problems, but they can help manage or reduce them. We consider proper nutrition a cornerstone in treating all health problems. Every year we get more scientific proof to support the old maxim: You are what you eat. That's why the first step toward improving attention and alertness should be the creation of a healthy diet. The recipes in this chapter will start you on that path.

STARTERS AND OTHER DELIGHTS

Grape Ice Cream Soda

2 cups Concord grape juice
2 cups club soda, chilled
4 scoops reduced-sugar vanilla ice cream

In a pitcher, combine the grape juice and club soda. Pour into 4 tall glasses. Top each with a scoop of vanilla ice cream.

Makes 4 servings

Recipe courtesy of the Concord Grape Association

Strawberry Smoothie

2 cups strawberries, hulled
1 cup milk
1¼ cups strawberry yogurt

In a blender, combine all the ingredients and blend on high speed until smooth. Pour into 4 glasses and serve immediately.

Makes 4 servings

Recipe courtesy of the Pioneer Valley Growers Association

"Walking" Apple Salad

1 large apple
1½ tablespoons peanut butter, any type
1 tablespoon raisins

Core the apple and remove the seeds. Scoop out part of the inside of apple with a small spoon and mix with the peanut butter and raisins in a small bowl. Stuff the mixture back into cored apple.

Makes 1 serving

Source: Bureau of Markets/Farmers' Markets

Spicy Hummus

2 tablespoons sesame seeds
2 tablespoons unsalted sunflower seeds
5 tablespoons canola oil
One 19-ounce can chickpeas, rinsed and drained
¼ cup fresh lemon juice
1 clove garlic, minced
½ teaspoon salt
1 teaspoon black pepper
Dash of cayenne pepper
¼ teaspoon curry powder
Cut-up fresh vegetables, pita crisps, or whole wheat crackers, to serve

In a food processor, combine the sesame seeds and sunflower seeds together. Add the oil and process until it forms a paste.

Add chickpeas to the mixture and process to break them down. Add the lemon juice, garlic, salt, black pepper, cayenne pepper, and curry powder and process until smooth. Place in a serving dish and serve with cut-up fresh vegetables, pita crisps, or whole wheat crackers.

Makes 2 servings

Recipe courtesy of the Manitoba Canola Growers Association

Creamy Peanut Dip

¼ cup creamy peanut butter, any type
2 tablespoons orange juice
½ cup lowfat vanilla yogurt
Fresh apple or pear slices and carrot or celery sticks, to serve

In a small bowl, mix the peanut butter and orange juice together until smooth. Stir in the yogurt, cover, and refrigerate until chilled. Serve with fresh apple or pear slices and carrot or celery sticks.

Makes 6 servings

Source: Food Stamp Nutrition Connection

SMART SIDE DISHES

Pinto Bean Salad

One 15-ounce can or 2 cups cooked pinto beans
1 cup diced celery
½ bunch green onions, finely sliced
1 tablespoon fresh or canned chopped green chiles (optional)
¾ cup shredded Colby, Monterey Jack, or cheddar cheese
¼ cup fat-free Thousand Island dressing
Salt
Lettuce leaves, to serve
Bacon bits, to garnish (optional)

Drain the pinto beans into a colander. In a serving bowl, combine the pinto beans, celery, green onions, chiles, if using, and cheese. Stir in the dressing to thoroughly coat, adding more dressing and salt if needed. Cover and refrigerate. Place lettuce leaves on 8 serving plates, top with the salad, and garnish with bacon bits, if using.

You can substitute mayonnaise or mayonnaise-type salad dressing for a milder salad.

You can substitute store-bought chili dressing for the Thousand Island dressing or add chili powder to the salad dressing and omit the green chiles to make a Chili Pinto Bean Salad.

Makes 8 servings

Recipe courtesy of the Northarvest Bean Growers Association

Luscious Lima Beans

Nonstick cooking spray
1 cup chopped celery
1 cup chopped onion
1 clove garlic, minced
1 cup chopped red bell pepper
One 10-ounce package frozen lima beans, thawed
One 10-ounce can chopped tomatoes with green chiles,
*   undrained*
1 cup low-sodium vegetable juice
1 teaspoon dried basil
1 bay leaf

Coat a large nonstick skillet with cooking spray and heat over medium until hot. Add the celery, onion, garlic, and bell pepper and sauté until tender-crisp, about 5 minutes. Add the remaining ingredients, stir well, and bring to boil. Cover, reduce the heat, and simmer until the lima beans are tender, about 8 to 10 minutes. Discard the bay leaf and serve.

Makes 4 to 6 servings

Source: Centers for Disease Control

Crunchy Greens

2 packed cups chopped spinach, collard greens, or beet greens
¼ cup finely diced onion
1 tablespoon water
¼ cup crunchy peanut butter, any type
1 small tomato, cut into wedges
Dash of black pepper
1 tablespoon soy sauce (optional)

In a medium saucepan, combine the spinach, onion, and water. Place over medium heat and cook, covered, for 3 to 5 minutes, or until the spinach is wilted. Add the peanut butter and tomato wedges and cook to heat through, 1 to 2 minutes longer. Add the pepper and the soy sauce, if using.

Makes 2 servings

Source: Bureau of Markets/Farmers' Markets

Skillet Summer Greens

¾ pound greens (Swiss chard, spinach, collard greens, or beet greens)
2 teaspoons vegetable oil
3 cloves garlic, minced, or ⅛ teaspoon garlic powder

Salt and black pepper
1 tablespoon apple cider vinegar

Coarsely chop the greens (including as much of the stems as possible). Heat a wok or large, heavy skillet over medium heat. Add the oil and heat it, then add the greens. Stir-fry for 3 to 5 minutes, until crisp-tender. Add the garlic and stir-fry for 2 minutes more. Transfer to a bowl. Sprinkle with salt and pepper to taste, then toss with the vinegar. Serve hot, cold, or at room temperature.

Makes 2 to 3 servings

Source: Bureau of Markets/Farmers Markets

Greens with Mango-Papaya Vinaigrette

1 large ripe mango, peeled, pitted, and diced
1 large papaya, peeled, seeded, and diced
⅓ cup canola oil
¼ cup apple cider vinegar
1 tablespoon honey
¼ teaspoon salt
½ teaspoon ground white pepper
8 lettuce leaves

Place the mango, papaya, oil, vinegar, honey, salt, and pepper in a food processor or blender. Process for 5 to 10 seconds, until smooth. Pour into a container and serve drizzled over lettuce leaves salad.

Makes 2 cups dressing and 8 servings

Recipe courtesy of the Hawaii Papaya Industry Association

Mashed Green Plantains

2 green or yellow plantains, peeled and cut in half
6 cups water
½ cup lowfat milk
5 tablespoons margarine
Salt and black pepper

In a medium saucepan, combine the plantains with the water and place over medium-high heat. Bring to a boil, cover, reduce the heat, and boil for 45 minutes, or until the plantains are soft. Drain; place the plantains in a medium bowl; add the milk, margarine, and salt and pepper to taste; and mash with an electric mixer or by hand. Serve as a side dish with any kind of meat, or substitute for mashed potatoes to liven up an ordinary meal.

Makes 4 servings

Recipe courtesy of the Turbana Corporation

Maggie's Squash Soup

1 small butternut squash
1 tablespoon canola oil
2 tablespoons water
4 ribs celery, chopped
2 medium leeks, white part only, cleaned and chopped
1 medium onion, chopped
Salt and black pepper
6 cups low-sodium chicken stock
1 cup lowfat milk or non-fat half and half
Warm toasted peanuts, to serve

Peel the squash and cut it into cubes. In a 5-quart saucepan, heat the oil and water over medium heat. Add the celery, leeks, and onion. Season with salt and pepper to taste and sauté for 5 minutes, or until softened. Add the squash and sauté for an additional 5 minutes, or until squash is soft. Add the chicken stock, raise the heat to medium-high, bring to a simmer, then reduce the heat and cook at a low simmer for 20 to 25 minutes. Season with salt and pepper to taste and remove the soup from the heat.

Transfer to a food processor and purée, then strain. Return the soup to the heat and bring to a simmer. Add the milk or half and half and heat to warm through. Portion the soup into warmed serving bowls and garnish with the peanuts.

Makes 8 servings

Recipe courtesy of Maggie Greenwood-Robinson

BRAIN POWER ENTRÉES

Beef Baked with Onions and Potatoes

1 pound lean ground beef
1 medium onion, chopped
4 large Russet potatoes, peeled and sliced
One 10½-ounce can vegetable-beef soup

Preheat the oven to 375°F. Lightly grease a medium-size casserole dish.

In a large skillet over medium-high heat, brown the ground beef and onions until the beef is no longer pink, then drain. Arrange the potato slices over the casserole. Spread the ground beef and onions over the potatoes. Pour the soup over the top. Cover with foil and bake for 45 minutes, then uncover and bake for another 25 minutes.

Makes 4 servings

Recipe courtesy of the Pioneer Valley Growers Association

Grilled Falafel Burgers

1 tablespoon olive oil, plus more for forming the patties
1 cup diced onion
1 tablespoon minced garlic
1 jalapeño or other green chile, seeded and minced
One 15-ounce can chickpeas, drained, or 1½ cups cooked
1 cup cooked and cooled basmati or other long-grain rice
1 tablespoon fresh lime juice
1¾ cups breadcrumbs
Salt and black pepper
Cayenne pepper or hot sauce
4 warmed pita pockets or toasted sandwich buns
Condiments of your choice (see recipe)
Tahini Mustard (recipe follows)

Heat the oil in a small skillet over medium heat. Add the onion and garlic and sauté until the onion is wilted and the garlic is golden. Add the jalapeño and stir well. Set aside to cool.

Place the cooled onion mixture, chickpeas, and rice in a food processor. Pulse on and off several times, until the mixture becomes a smooth puree. Transfer to a large bowl. Add the lime juice and 1 cup of the breadcrumbs. Season with salt, black pepper, and cayenne to taste.

Spread some oil over your hands and shape the mixture into four 3-inch patties that are ½ inch thick. Add the reserved breadcrumbs if the patties don't hold their shape. They should be slightly sticky.

Prepare a grill or preheat the broiler. Place the patties on a fine-mesh seafood or vegetable grid and grill about 5 inches from the heat for 4 to 6 minutes per side, or until lightly browned, checking often so they don't burn.

Tuck the patties into warmed pita pockets or toasted sandwich buns along with shredded lettuce, tomato slices, sweet onion slices, alfalfa sprouts, and a dollop of Tahini Mustard.

Makes 4 servings

Tahini Mustard

¼ *cup tahini*
¼ *cup Dijon-style mustard, plus more if needed*
¼ *cup fresh lime juice*
1 *tablespoon minced garlic*
¾ *cup water*

Place all the ingredients in a blender and blend until smooth. Taste and add up to 1 tablespoon additional mustard, if desired. The mustard can be stored tightly covered in the refrigerator for several days.

Makes ½ cup

Recipe courtesy of Andrea Landate

Southwestern Bean Burgers

1 cup canned white kidney beans, rinsed, drained, and mashed
1 cup mild prepared salsa
½ cup plain dried breadcrumbs
1 tablespoon minced fresh cilantro or flat-leaf parsley
Dash of hot sauce
Nonstick cooking spray
¾ ounce reduced-fat shredded cheddar cheese

In a medium bowl, combine the beans, ½ cup of the salsa, the breadcrumbs, cilantro, and hot sauce. Using your hands, shape into 4 equal-size patties. Place the patties on a large plate, cover with plastic, and refrigerate for 20 minutes, or until firm.

Spray a 12-inch nonstick skillet with cooking spray and heat over medium heat. Add the patties and cook for about 5 minutes on each side, or until browned.

To serve, top the patties with the remaining salsa and the cheese.

Makes 2 servings

Recipe courtesy of Andrea Laudate

Lentil Patties with Walnut Sauce

LENTIL PATTIES
1 cup canned lentils, rinsed and drained
¼ cup seasoned dry breadcrumbs
1 large egg white
1 clove garlic, minced
Nonstick cooking spray

WALNUT SAUCE

1 teaspoon margarine

¼ cup finely chopped onion

1½ teaspoons all-purpose flour

½ cup lowfat milk

¼ cup minced fresh parsley

2 tablespoons finely chopped walnuts

Dash of ground nutmeg

In a medium bowl, use a fork to slightly mash the lentils. Add the breadcrumbs, egg white, and garlic and mix well. Shape into 4 equal-size patties.

Spray a 12-inch nonstick skillet with cooking spray and heat over medium-high heat. Add the patties and cook for about 4 minutes on each side, or until browned. Transfer the patties to a serving platter. Cover with foil to keep warm.

In the same skillet over high heat, melt the margarine, then add the onion and cook, stirring frequently, for about 1 minute, or until slightly softened.

Reduce the heat to medium. Sprinkle the flour over the onion and stir quickly to combine. Cook for another minute, stirring constantly. Slowly stir in the milk, then add the parsley, walnuts, and nutmeg. Cook for about 2 minutes, stirring frequently, until the mixture thickens. Serve the lentil patties topped with the walnut sauce.

Makes 2 servings

Recipe courtesy of Andrea Laudate

Beef Stroganoff

1 pound lean beef (top round)
2 teaspoons vegetable oil
¼ cup finely chopped onion
1 pound button mushrooms, sliced
¼ teaspoon salt
Black pepper
¼ teaspoon ground nutmeg
½ teaspoon dried basil
¼ cup white wine
1 cup lowfat plain yogurt
6 cups cooked macaroni

Cut the beef into 1-inch cubes. In a nonstick skillet, heat 1 teaspoon of the oil over medium heat. Add the onion and sauté for 2 minutes, or until softened. Add the beef, raise the heat to medium-high, and cook for an additional 5 minutes, or until evenly browned. Remove the beef from the pan and add the remaining 1 teaspoon oil to the pan. Reduce the heat to medium and add the mushrooms. Sauté until softened, about 5 minutes. Add the beef and onions to the pan, along with the salt, pepper to taste, nutmeg, and basil. Add the wine and yogurt and stir gently. Heat the mixture through, but do not bring to a boil. Spoon the macaroni into serving bowls and serve the beef on top.

Makes 4 to 6 servings

Source: U.S. Department of Health and Human Services

Chicken Marsala

¼ teaspoon salt
⅛ teaspoon black pepper
¼ cup all-purpose flour
Four 5-ounce boneless, skinless chicken breasts
1 tablespoon olive oil
½ cup Marsala wine
Juice of ½ lemon
½ cup low-sodium chicken broth
½ cup sliced button mushrooms
1 tablespoon chopped fresh parsley

On a large plate, mix together the salt, pepper, and flour and spread it over the plate. Coat the chicken on all sides with the seasoned flour. In a heavy-bottomed skillet over medium-high heat, heat the oil. Place the chicken breasts in the skillet and brown on both sides. Remove the chicken from the skillet and set aside on a plate. Add the wine to the skillet and stir until the wine is heated. Add the lemon juice, broth, and mushrooms. Stir to combine, then reduce the heat and cook for about 10 minutes, or until the sauce is partially reduced. Return the browned chicken breasts to the skillet, spooning the sauce over the chicken. Cover and cook for 5 to 10 minutes, until the chicken is cooked through. Transfer the chicken to serving plates and spoon the sauce over the chicken. Garnish with the parsley.

Makes 4 servings

Source: U.S. Department of Health and Human Services

Chicken and Spanish Rice

2 teaspoons vegetable oil
1 cup chopped onions
¼ cup chopped green bell peppers
One 8-ounce can prepared tomato sauce
1 teaspoon chopped fresh parsley
1¼ teaspoons minced garlic
½ teaspoon black pepper
5 cups cooked brown rice
3½ cups diced, cooked chicken breasts

In a large skillet, heat the oil over medium heat. Add the onions and bell peppers and sauté for 5 minutes, or until softened. Add the tomato sauce, parsley, garlic, and black pepper and cook to heat through. Add the cooked rice and chicken and cook to heat through.

Makes 6 servings

Source: U.S. Department of Health and Human Services

Scallop Kabobs

3 medium green bell peppers, cut into 1½-inch squares
1½ pounds fresh bay scallops
1 pint cherry tomatoes
¼ cup dry white wine
¼ cup vegetable oil
3 tablespoons fresh lemon juice
Dash of garlic powder
Black pepper

Preheat a grill or the broiler.

In a medium pot of boiling water, parboil the bell peppers for 2 minutes. Drain and cool. Thread the bell peppers, scallops, and cherry tomatoes onto 4 skewers, alternating the ingredients. In a medium bowl, whisk together the wine, oil, lemon juice, garlic powder, and black pepper to taste. Brush the kabobs with the marinade. Place on the grill or under the broiler and grill for 15 minutes, turning and basting frequently, until scallops are cooked through.

Makes 4 servings

Source: U.S. Department of Health and Human Services

ENERGIZING DESSERTS

Pumpkin Pie

One 16-ounce can pure pumpkin
One 12-ounce can sweetened condensed milk
2 large eggs
1 teaspoon pumpkin pie spice
1 prebaked 9-inch pie shell
Reduced-sugar vanilla ice cream or whipped topping, to serve

Preheat the oven to 425°F.

In a large bowl, combine the pumpkin, condensed milk, eggs, and pumpkin pie spice and whisk together. Pour into the pie shell and bake for 15 minutes, then reduce the heat to 350°F and bake for 35 to 40 minutes longer, or until a knife inserted near the center comes out clean. Remove from the oven and cool on a wire rack. Serve with scoops of reduced-sugar vanilla ice cream or whipped topping.

Makes 8 to 10 servings

Recipe courtesy of the Pioneer Valley Growers Association

Easy Fruitcake

3 cups whole Brazil nuts, shelled and pulverized in a blender after measuring

2 cups dates, pitted

1 cup dried unsweetened cherries

¾ cup all-purpose flour

¾ cup sugar

½ teaspoon baking powder

½ teaspoon salt

3 large eggs, beaten

1 teaspoon vanilla extract

Preheat the oven to 300°F. Grease a 9½×5½×2½-inch baking pan and line with wax paper.

In a large bowl, combine the Brazil nuts, dates, and cherries. In a separate bowl, combine the flour, sugar, baking powder, and salt. Sift the dry ingredients over the fruit and nut mixture and mix well until fully coated. In a medium bowl, beat the eggs until foamy and add the vanilla. Stir into the fruit mixture. Turn the mixture into the baking pan and spread evenly. Bake for 1 hour and 45 minutes, or until cake is firm to the touch.

Remove to a wire rack to cool completely before cutting. Wrap with plastic wrap and store in the refrigerator.

Makes 8 to 10 servings

Recipe courtesy of Maggie Greenwood-Robinson

Black Bean Brownies

Nonstick cooking spray
½ cup unsalted butter or margarine, softened
2 cups sugar
½ cup unsweetened cocoa powder
1 cup cooked black beans, drained and puréed in a blender
4 large eggs
⅔ cup all-purpose flour
½ teaspoon baking powder
1 teaspoon salt
chocolate frosting (optional)

Preheat the oven to 350°F. Coat a 9×13-inch baking pan with cooking spray.

In a large bowl, mix together the butter, sugar, cocoa, black bean puree, and eggs until well blended. In a separate bowl, sift together the flour, baking powder, and salt and stir into the wet ingredients. Pour the batter into the baking pan and bake for 40 minutes, or until knife inserted in center comes out clean. If you like, frost with your favorite chocolate frosting, or any canned chocolate frosting.

Recipe courtesy of the Northarvest Bean Growers Association

Sweet Plantains in Cranberry Syrup

3 very ripe plantains
1 cup unsweetened cranberry juice
½ cup brown sugar
1 cinnamon stick
Reduced-sugar vanilla ice cream or whipped cream, to serve

Peel the plantains and cut into thin rounds. Place in a small saucepan and add the cranberry juice, brown sugar, and cinnamon stick. Place over medium-high heat, bring to a boil, then lower the heat and simmer for about 2 hours, stirring every 30 minutes, until mixture is thick and plantains are soft.

To make in the microwave, cut the ends off the unpeeled plantains and place the plantains on a microwave-safe plate. Place a moist paper towel over them and microwave on high for about 8 minutes, or until the skin opens up. Let cool, then peel. Slice into thin rounds and place in a microwave-safe baking dish. Add the cranberry juice, brown sugar, and cinnamon stick. Microwave on high for 2 to 3 minutes, or until mixture is heated through. Serve with reduced-sugar vanilla ice cream or whipped cream.

Recipe courtesy of the Turbana Corporation

Granola Bars

1 cup honey
1 cup chunky peanut butter, any kind
3½ cups rolled oats
½ cup raisins
½ cup grated carrot
½ cup unsweetened flaked coconut

Preheat the oven to 350°F.

In a large saucepan, over low heat, combine the honey and peanut butter until they melt. Remove the pan from the heat. Add the oats, raisins, carrot, and coconut to the saucepan. Stir well, and let the mixture cool in the saucepan until you can safely touch it with your hands. Transfer the mixture to a 9×13-inch baking pan and press firmly into the bottom of the pan. Bake for 25 minutes, or until bars are slightly browned. Cool before cutting.

Makes 24 bars

Source: Food Stamp Nutrition Connection

SMART TIPS ⚫ BOOST YOUR POWERS OF CONCENTRATION

- Breathe in long cycles that emphasize the inhalation phase.

- Chew sugarless gum: it enhances concentration.

- Set periods of time, such as twenty minutes at a time, in which you will concentrate on something, such as reading a book or maga-zine.

- Take breaks when needed. If you get upset or feel overstimulated, it will break your concentration. Give yourself a time-out. Leave the situation or go to a quiet place to calm down.

- Make lists and computerized schedules to help you better organize your life and set priorities.

- Break down projects into small, manageable steps.

- Reflect a 25-watt blue light on your work area—it helps the brain focus.

continued

- Reduce distractions by removing clutter from your desk.

- Listen to rhythmic music, as research shows that it boosts blood flow to the brain. Increased blood flow aids in concentration, memory, and other mental tasks.

- Exercise regularly, as exercise channels oxygen to the brain to keep it alert. It also relieves stress, works off aggression, and energizes the body.

FIVE

※

Memory-Boosting Meals

If you could get a glimpse of your life at seventy or eighty, wouldn't it be nice to see yourself as mentally sharp as you are today? Some good news: Your mind does not have to turn to mush as you age, as long as you take care of your brain now. You can boost your brain power and keep your memory intact well into your golden years by living a healthier lifestyle. More than any organ in your body, your brain relies on a minute-to-minute supply of nutrients for peak functioning. The right foods can have an enormous impact on your memory, and you can bring back a faltering memory by populating your diet with the right choices.

You don't have to wait until you reach your golden years to enhance your memory. Your capacity to store information is the most important aspect of cognitive functioning in your job or in school. These functions apply whether you are four or a hundred and four. Parents should be very alert to how their children's grades can be affected by food ingredients. Teens need their memories to be sharp every day because their brains are in the process of being pruned for specialized skills. In fact, they will be having enormous problems in judgment, regardless of how smart they are, and they can use all the memory power they can get in times of critical choices.

As a general rule of thumb, be sure to follow a nutritious diet, devoid of highly processed foods, to supply your brain with the nutrients and energy it needs for optimal functioning and psychological health. A memory-boosting diet is one that includes at least five servings of fruits and vegetables daily, several servings of whole grains, moderate amounts of lean proteins (fish, poultry, lean red meat, and dairy products), and some fat. Beyond these basics, certain foods have emerged as champion memory boosters for unmuddling your mind and enhancing your recall. Take a look.

Sip Green Tea

Drinking green tea is recommended for memory preservation. It protects against cognitive decline in the elderly by reducing bodily levels of cholesterol and homocysteine, a harmful protein that has been implicated in heart disease. Both substances are associated with beta-amyloid peptides, proteins forming the plaques that clog the brains of Alzheimer's sufferers. If this disease strikes, you gradually lose your mind, your memory, and the ability to recognize your loved ones. In the advanced stages of the disease, you become totally dependent on others for your care. An antioxidant in green tea called epigallocatechin-3-gallate (EGCG) is believed to decrease production of these proteins.

Put More Fish on Your Dish

When I (Frank) was completing my internship at New York Medical Center, I was on a very limited budget. Scrimping and saving, I allotted only one dollar a day for my lunches, which meant that I had to either save up for a sandwich a week or find some pretty cheap food. I tried the candy bars in the vending machine, with disastrous results. Not only did I get hungrier, but I temporarily lost some intellectual skills. Then I made a discovery—sardines. The cost at that time was twenty-five cents a can, and I could get all the crackers I wanted from the cafeteria. You may think that I would have gotten tired of eating those little fishes every day, but I felt stronger and less hungry. And I lost twenty-five pounds as an added benefit. Most important, I could recite the whole dictionary of psychological protocols. My mental recall was operating at peak condition.

It bears repeating that fish is good for everything brain-related, and memory is no exception. Fish is loaded with super-healthy fats called omega-3 fatty acids, which are vital for optimum brain health. Plenty of scientific evidence reveals that omega-3 fats combat depression, improve intellectual performance, rebuild the fatty membranes of brain cells, and protect against stroke. A series of strokes can cause a form of memory loss called multi-infarct dementia (also called vascular dementia) that leaves pockets of dead brain tissue (infarcts). The accumulated effect of these strokes can lead to gradual loss of memory.

A good antistroke measure is to eat two or three fish meals a week. Include tuna or oysters in some of these fish meals. Both are loaded with zinc, a mineral that plays a vital role in memory formation and retention. What if you don't like fish? Include walnuts in your diet. They're packed with omega-3 fats, too.

Fill Up on Antioxidant-Rich Fruits and Veggies

Remember that your brain is highly vulnerable to oxidation, a tissue-damaging process that occurs when oxygen reacts with fat. The by-products of this reaction are devilish molecules called free radicals that attack bodily tissues and damage your memory and mental faculties over time.

Fortunately, though, oxidation and the free radicals it produces can be neutralized by antioxidants, available from food and supplements, and found naturally in the body. The chief vitamin antioxidants are vitamin C, vitamin E, and beta-carotene; the chief mineral antioxidants are selenium, copper, zinc, and manganese. As we've emphasized, the best way to increase your supply of antioxidants is to eat plenty of fruits and vegetables every day. Include a variety of green, orange, yellow, and purple fruits and vegetables in your diet for maximum antioxidant power.

Fruits and veggies are also loaded with antistroke nutrients. Folic acid is one of them, because it prevents the buildup of homocysteine in your body. Another stroke-preventive nutrient in these foods is potassium. Not getting enough potassium in your diet can increase your chance of stroke by 50 percent. Potassium is plentiful in bananas, potatoes, avocados, lima beans, tomatoes, spinach, and oranges.

Make Your Memory Stay with Some Blueberries Each Day

Eating blueberries as a regular part of your diet may squelch the loss of short-term memory that occurs with age, according to a Tufts University study conducted with rats. Much like people, rats become more forgetful as they get older. For two months, the researchers supplemented their subjects' diets with the human equivalent of 1 cup of blueberries daily. Compared with rats that did not eat the fruit, the blueberry-fed rats showed improvements in their memory performance. If the fruit proves to have the same effect on humans, reversing short-term memory loss could be as easy as devoting between 1 percent and 2 percent of your daily diet to blueberries. It isn't clear how blueberries confer their benefits, but presumably some of the antioxidants that produce the blue color also protect cells against cell-damaging free radicals.

With these foods in mind, here are some easy-to-fix recipes that will help you fend off fuzzy thinking. Each recipe contains nutrients proven to improve memory-linked brain chemistry and protect against memory loss.

SMART TIPS ● FIVE SURPRISING WAYS TO BOOST YOUR MEMORY

USE IT OR LOSE IT. Your brain cells communicate with each other through fiberlike branches called dendrites. When brain cells are stimulated, dendrites grow, increasing the number of connections between cells. This improves your memory, attention span, and ability

continued

to learn. One of the best ways to build new connections is to use your brain. Some suggestions: learn a language, solve crossword puzzles, do a jigsaw puzzle, memorize Bible verses or poetry, learn a musical instrument, or become a tutor. And numerous studies show that people who regularly challenge their body and brain are less likely to lose cognitive function later in life—and may even reduce their chances of getting Alzheimer's disease.

STAY EDUCATED. Research has found that having an intellectually challenging occupation or more education helps you stay mentally sharp as you get older—and may even be protective against the development of Alzheimer's disease.

MANAGE STRESS. When you're persistently stressed out or depressed, your adrenal glands churn out stress hormones. If stress is chronic, these hormones stay elevated, inflicting damage to the brain by destroying cells in the hippocampus, the seahorse-shaped structure deep within the brain that helps you learn and remember. Some ideas for getting stress under control: Learn how to relax, pursue recreational activities, exercise, simplify your life, or undergo counseling to reprogram your reaction to stress-provoking events.

SLEEP WELL. Bad sleep damages memory and learning ability, and scientists believe that memory loss attributed to old age may be related to poor sleep. In addition to the standard good-sleep advice like maintaining a regular sleep schedule, it's important to keep your room well ventilated, eliminate sleep-robbing substances such as caffeine and alcohol, sleep on a mattress that is supportive and comfortable, exercise regularly, and eat a nutritious diet.

MARRY SMART. Being married to a smart spouse helps prevent mental decline. That's the finding of research demonstrating that people who marry smart are more likely to retain their intellectual abilities as they age.

BELIEVE YOU HAVE A GOOD MEMORY. What you believe about your memory helps you remember better, says a study conducted at the University of Florida in Gainesville. Volunteers who were told that memory was a skill that could be improved (it can) performed better on a difficult memory task than those who were told otherwise. The lesson here: Stop telling yourself you're forgetful, or forgetfulness could become a self-fulfilling prophecy. The sky's the limit when you think you can.

STARTERS AND OTHER DELIGHTS

Green Tea Smoothie

1 cup green tea, chilled
2 cups diced honeydew melon
2 kiwis, peeled and diced
1 banana
1 tablespoon cane sugar
Dash of salt
6 ice cubes

In a food processor, combine all the ingredients and process until smooth. Pour into tall glasses and serve immediately.

Makes 2 servings

Recipe courtesy of Wholesome Sweeteners

Blue Hawaii Smoothie

2¼ cups frozen blueberries
8 ice cubes
2 cups pineapple juice
1 banana

In blender, combine all the ingredients and blend until smooth. Pour into glasses and serve immediately.

Makes 4 servings

Recipe courtesy of the Michigan Blueberry Growers Association

Glazed Blueberry Breakfast Rolls

Nonstick cooking spray
One 10-ounce can refrigerated pizza crust dough
All-purpose flour, for rolling the dough

BLUEBERRY FILLING
¾ cup blueberries, finely chopped
2 tablespoons orange juice
2 tablespoons granulated sugar
2 teaspoons cornstarch
1 teaspoon grated orange zest

GLAZE
½ cup powdered sugar
1 tablespoon milk
½ teaspoon grated orange zest

Preheat the oven to 375°F. Coat 12 muffin cups with cooking spray.

In a small saucepan, combine the blueberry filling ingredients, stirring to dissolve the cornstarch. Place over medium heat and cook, stirring constantly, until thick and bubbly, about 3 minutes. Remove from the heat and set aside to cool for 10 minutes. Unroll the pizza dough onto a lightly floured surface and pat into a 12×9-inch rectangle. Spread the blueberry filling over the dough, leaving a ½-inch border along the sides. Beginning with a long side, roll up jelly-roll fashion and pinch the seam to seal (do not seal the ends of the roll). Cut the roll into twelve 1-inch slices. Place the slices, cut sides up, in the muffin cups. Bake for 12 to 15 minutes, until lightly browned. Remove the rolls from the pan, and cool on a wire rack for at least 15 minutes before glazing.

To make the glaze, in a small bowl, combine the powdered sugar, milk, and orange zest, stirring until smooth. Drizzle the icing over the rolls.

Makes 12 rolls

Recipe courtesy of the Michigan Blueberry Growers Association

Fruit Salad Parfait

1 cup lowfat vanilla yogurt
½ cup sliced peaches, apples, pears, or other fruit
½ cup strawberries, blueberries, or other berries
Granola or graham crackers, for topping (optional)

Spoon ¼ cup yogurt into each of 2 glasses. Add half of the fruit to each glass. Top each with ¼ cup yogurt. Finish with granola or crushed graham crackers, if using.

Makes 2 servings

Source: Bureau of Markets/Farmers' Markets

Southwest Spiced Walnuts

2 cups walnut halves and pieces
1 tablespoon sugar
1 teaspoon sea salt
½ teaspoon garlic powder
¼ teaspoon ground cumin
½ teaspoon cayenne pepper
1 tablespoon walnut oil or canola oil

Preheat the oven to 350°F.

Spread the walnuts over a baking sheet and toast in the oven for 10 minutes. Remove from the oven and cool.

In a small bowl, mix together the sugar, salt, garlic powder, cumin, and cayenne. Heat the oil in a large skillet over medium heat. Add the toasted walnuts and toss for 1 minute. Add the seasoning mixture and toss until the walnuts are coated. Transfer to paper towels to cool.

Makes 2 cups

Recipe courtesy of the Walnut Marketing Board

SMART SIDE DISHES

Summer Fruit Salad

1 cup diced fresh or frozen strawberries
1 cup cubed watermelon
1 cup pineapple chunks (fresh or canned packed in natural
    juice)

In a medium bowl, combine the fruit. Cover and chill.

Makes 4 servings

Source: Food Stamp Nutrition Connection

Parsnip, Tomato, and Cheese Casserole

1½ pounds parsnips
1 medium onion
1 cup cooked orzo or other small pasta
One 14-ounce can whole tomatoes with juices
1 cup grated part-skim mozzarella cheese
Freshly grated nutmeg, for dusting
⅔ cup nonfat plain yogurt

Preheat the oven to 375°F.

Cut the parsnips and onion into thin slices. Scatter half the pasta over a 9-inch ovenproof dish. Layer half the onions, parsnips, and tomatoes on top. Sprinkle with half the cheese and dust with nutmeg. Repeat the layers and spread the yogurt over the top. Cover with foil and bake for 30 minutes. Remove the cover and bake for 5 to 10 minutes more, or until the top is crisp and browned.

Makes 4 servings

Recipe courtesy of Andrea Laudate

Potato, Pepper, and Onion Bake

1 pound Russet potatoes (about 3 medium)
1 to 1½ pounds bell peppers (4 medium, green, yellow, orange, and/or red)

1 large sweet onion
2 tablespoons vegetable oil
Black pepper

Preheat the oven to 425°F.

Cut the potatoes into 1-inch chunks. (Peel thick-skinned potatoes.) Cut the bell peppers into 2-inch pieces. Cut the onion into chunks. Place the potatoes, bell peppers, and onions in a shallow ovenproof dish. Pour the oil over the vegetables and lightly toss to coat with the oil. Sprinkle with black pepper. Bake for 30 minutes.

Makes 4 servings

Source: Bureau of Markets/Farmers' Markets

The Best Carrot Salad in the History of the Universe

2 pounds carrots, shredded
10 to 14 ounces cranberry lemonade, depending on how juicy
     you like your salad
1 cup dried unsweetened cranberries
1 cup golden raisins
1 cup coarsely chopped walnuts
1/3 cup sesame seeds
Juice and pulp of 1 lemon
1 to 2 teaspoons orange flower water, to taste

Soak the dried fruit in the lemonade to soften a bit if you like. In a large bowl, combine all the ingredients and toss. Refrigerate and serve cool.

Makes 20 servings

Recipe courtesy of Andrea Laudate

Mashed Sweet Potatoes

4 tablespoons unsalted butter, cut into 4 pieces
2 tablespoons heavy cream
1 teaspoon sugar
½ teaspoon salt
2 pounds (2 to 3 large) sweet potatoes, peeled and quartered
Black pepper

In a medium saucepan, combine the butter, heavy cream, sugar, salt, and sweet potatoes. Place over low heat and cook, covered, for 35 to 45 minutes, or until the sweet potatoes fall apart when poked with a fork. Remove from the heat. Mash the sweet potatoes directly in the saucepan with a potato masher and transfer to warmed serving bowls. Sprinkle with pepper and serve immediately.

Makes 4 servings

Source: Food Stamp Nutrition Connection

Red, White, and Green Salad

½ small head cauliflower
1 small head broccoli
1 medium tomato, chopped
¼ medium red onion, sliced
3 to 4 tablespoons reduced-fat Italian dressing

Break off the tops of the cauliflower and broccoli and chop the stems. Steam or microwave the tops and stems until crisp-tender.

Place the cauliflower, broccoli, tomato, and onion in a salad bowl. Add the dressing, toss gently, and serve.

Makes 3 to 4 servings

Source: Bureau of Markets/Farmers' Markets

Vegetable Fried Rice

2 teaspoons vegetable oil
½ cup sliced celery
¼ cup chopped onion
¼ teaspoon garlic powder or 1 clove garlic, minced
¼ cup peas
¼ cup chopped carrot
¼ cup corn or chopped broccoli, bell peppers, or mushrooms
  (optional)
2 cups cooked rice
1 tablespoon Worcestershire sauce or soy sauce
Dash of black pepper

In a wok or large skillet, heat the oil. Add the celery, onion, and garlic and stir-fry for 2 minutes, or until crisp-tender. Add the peas, carrots, and corn, if using. Stir-fry for about 4 minutes, or until the vegetables are tender, stirring constantly. Add the rice, Worcestershire sauce, and pepper and stir-fry for about 2 minutes, to heat through. Serve immediately.

Makes 4 servings

Source: Food Stamp Nutrition Connection

Walnut Crunch Couscous

1 tablespoon olive oil
¾ cup chopped walnuts
1 small clove garlic, minced or pressed
½ cup lightly packed chopped fresh mint
½ cup lightly packed chopped fresh cilantro
½ teaspoon coarse salt
2 cups low-sodium vegetable broth, chicken broth, or water
1 cup uncooked couscous

Heat the oil in a medium skillet over medium heat. Add the walnuts and cook, stirring, until lightly toasted and fragrant, about 4 minutes. Add the garlic and cook for 1 minute. Remove from the heat and let cool. Toss with the mint and cilantro.

In a medium saucepan over high heat, bring the broth to a boil. Add the couscous. Remove from heat, cover, and let stand for 5 minutes. Fluff with a fork and stir in walnut-herb mixture.

Makes 4 servings

Recipe courtesy of the Walnut Marketing Board

Oven-Cooked Green Tea Rice

2 cups boiling water
8 green tea bags
1 tablespoon unsalted butter
1 cup uncooked long-grain rice
½ teaspoon salt

Preheat the oven to 350°F.

Combine the boiling water and green tea bags. Let stand for 10 minutes, then remove the tea bags.

In a 1-quart casserole dish, combine the green tea and butter; stir until the butter melts. Stir in the rice and salt. Cover the casserole and bake for 30 to 35 minutes, until the rice is tender and the liquid is absorbed. Fluff with a fork, and serve.

Makes 4 servings

Recipe courtesy of R.C. Bigelow

BRAIN POWER ENTRÉES

Tarragon-Walnut Chicken Salad

4 boneless, skinless chicken breast halves

¼ cup mayonnaise

¼ cup sour cream

1 tablespoon tarragon wine vinegar

½ teaspoon salt

⅛ teaspoon freshly ground black pepper

2 tablespoons walnut oil

2 tablespoons chopped fresh tarragon, plus 4 small sprigs

1 tablespoon chopped fresh chives

1 cup chopped walnuts

½ cup chopped dried apricots

4 large lettuce leaves

Place the chicken in a large skillet or Dutch oven. Add enough water to cover the chicken. Bring to a gentle boil over medium-high heat. Reduce the heat to low and simmer for 15 minutes, or until no longer pink in the center and the juices run clear. Remove the chicken from the liquid. Cool and cut into ½-inch cubes.

In a small bowl, blend together the mayonnaise and sour cream, then stir in the vinegar, salt, and pepper. Whisk in the oil until blended. Stir in the tarragon and chives. Reserve 2 tablespoons of the walnuts and 2 tablespoons of the apricots for garnish, and add the remainder to the dressing. Mix well. Stir in the chicken, cover, and refrigerate for 1 to 2 hours, until well chilled.

Place 1 lettuce leaf on each of 4 plates and mound the chicken salad onto the leaves.

Makes 4 servings

Recipe courtesy of Andrea Laudate

Tuna Quesadillas

Two 6-ounce cans water-packed tuna, drained
1 tablespoon reduced-fat mayonnaise
4 flour tortillas
½ cup grated reduced-fat cheddar cheese
Nonstick cooking spray (if cooking on the stovetop)

In a small bowl, mix the tuna with the mayonnaise.

To make in the microwave, spoon the tuna onto one half of each tortilla. Top with the cheese and fold the tortillas in half. Place on plates and microwave on high for 60 seconds, turning the plates halfway through cooking time.

To make on the stovetop, divide the tuna between 2 of the tortillas. Sprinkle with the cheese and top with the remaining 2 tortillas.

Spray a medium skillet with cooking spray. One at a time, cook the quesadillas on both sides, until browned and the cheese is melted. Cut in half and serve.

Makes 4 servings

Source: Food Stamp Nutrition Connection

Herbed Baked Fish

1 pound salmon or any type of whitefish, fresh or frozen
¼ teaspoon paprika
¼ teaspoon garlic powder
¼ teaspoon onion powder
⅛ teaspoon black pepper
⅛ teaspoon dried oregano
⅛ teaspoon dried thyme
1 tablespoon fresh lemon juice
1½ tablespoons margarine, melted

If using frozen fish, thaw in the refrigerator according to package directions. Preheat the oven to 350°F.

Separate or cut the fish into 4 pieces. Place the fish in a 9×13×2-inch baking pan. In a small bowl, combine the paprika, garlic powder, onion powder, black pepper, oregano, and thyme. Sprinkle the herb mixture and lemon juice evenly over the fish, then drizzle the melted margarine on top. Bake for 20 to 25 minutes, until the fish flakes easily with a fork. Serve immediately.

Makes 4 servings

Source: U.S. Department of Agriculture

Salmon Patties

One 15½-ounce can salmon, drained
1 cup crushed whole grain cereal or crackers
2 large eggs, lightly beaten
½ cup lowfat milk
⅛ teaspoon black pepper
1 tablespoon vegetable oil

Use a fork or clean fingers to flake salmon until very fine. Place in a large bowl and add the cereal, eggs, milk, and black pepper. Mix thoroughly. Shape into 8 patties. Heat the oil in a large skillet over medium heat. Carefully cook the patties on both sides until thoroughly cooked and browned, about 6 to 8 minutes on each side.

Makes 8 servings

Note: You can substitute canned tuna for the salmon, or make a combination of the two.

Source: Food Stamp Nutrition Connection

Blueberry-Stuffed Cornish Game Hens

8 Cornish game hens
Salt and black pepper
¼ cup vegetable oil
¼ cup fresh lemon juice
¼ cup angostura bitters
4 cups fresh blueberries
4 teaspoons sugar
½ cup unsalted butter or margarine, softened
8 small bay leaves

Preheat the oven to 350°F.

Sprinkle the game hens inside and out with salt and pepper. In a small bowl, whisk together the oil, lemon juice, and angostura bitters, and brush the game hens with the mixture, inside and out. Fill each bird with ½ cup blueberries and ½ teaspoon sugar. Sew or skewer the opening and place in a shallow roasting pan. Spread the butter over the breasts of the birds and place a bay leaf on top. Roast for 1 hour, or until a leg is easily moved.

Remove from the oven and serve.

Makes 8 servings

Recipe courtesy of the Michigan Blueberry Growers Association

ENERGIZING DESSERTS

Blueberry Fruit Leather

4 cups fresh blueberries
1 cup fresh strawberries, hulled
¼ cup honey
1 tablespoon almond extract

Place the blueberries and strawberries in blender or food processor and blend until smooth. Press the mixture through a strainer into a bowl to remove the skin and seeds. Stir in the honey and almond extract. Place mixture in a large skillet over very low heat. Cook, stirring frequently, for 1 hour, or until thickened.

Preheat the oven to 150°F. Line a cookie sheet with parchment paper (or foil). Pour the thickened fruit mixture onto the cookie sheet and spread to form an 8×12-inch rectangle. Bake for 5½ to 6 hours, until the fruit sheet is dry enough so that it doesn't stick to your fingers but moist enough to roll. You can place a potholder in the oven door to keep it ajar—this will help dry the leather by allowing moisture to escape. Remove from the oven, cool, and cut into 3×4-inch squares. Store in an air-tight container or rolled in plastic wrap.

Makes 6 pieces

Recipe courtesy of the Michigan Blueberry Growers Association

Fresh Blueberry-Strawberry Mousse Pie

1 envelope unflavored gelatin
¼ cup cold water
2 tablespoons fresh lemon juice
1 cup fresh blueberries, finely chopped, plus whole blueberries to garnish
1 cup hulled sliced fresh strawberries, finely chopped, plus sliced strawberries to garnish
¾ cup confectioners' sugar
One 8-ounce container light whipped topping, plus more to garnish
One 9-inch prepared graham cracker crumb pie crust
Blueberry Sauce (recipe follows)

In a small saucepan, sprinkle the gelatin over the cold water; let stand 1 minute. Place over low heat and stir until the gelatin is completely dissolved, about 1 minute. Stir in the lemon juice and set aside to cool.

In a large bowl, combine the blueberries, strawberries, and confectioners' sugar, and toss to coat. Stir in the dissolved gelatin. Fold in the whipped topping, and spoon the filling into the crust. Cover directly with plastic and refrigerate for 3 to 4 hours, until firm. Garnish with whipped topping, fresh fruit, and Blueberry Sauce.

Makes 8 servings

Blueberry Sauce

2 cups fresh or frozen and thawed blueberries
¼ cup orange juice
¼ cup water
¼ cup sugar
1 tablespoon cornstarch

In a medium saucepan, combine all the ingredients. Place over medium heat and cook, stirring constantly, for 4 to 5 minutes, until thickened.

Cool before spooning onto the Fresh Blueberry-Strawberry Mousse Pie.

Makes 2 cups

Recipe courtesy of the Michigan Blueberry Growers Association

Grapefruit Granita

2 cups pink grapefruit juice
¼ cup sugar
4 mint leaves
4 pink grapefruit slices

In a medium saucepan, combine the grapefruit juice and sugar. Bruise the mint leaves between your fingers and add to the saucepan. Place over medium heat and bring the mixture just to a boil, stirring to dissolve the sugar. Remove from the heat, cover, and let stand 5 minutes. Remove the mint leaves.

Pour the grapefruit juice mixture into ice cube trays and freeze. Just before serving, place a single layer of frozen cubes in a food processor. Pulse 12 times, or until no large chunks of ice remain. Repeat with the remaining cubes. Spoon the granita into 4 stemmed glasses. Garnish each with a grapefruit slice. Serve immediately.

Makes 4 servings

Recipe courtesy of the Florida Department of Citrus Headquarters

Orange Custard Pie

1¼ cups orange juice
1 cup skim milk
2 large egg yolks
½ cup sugar
3 tablespoons cornstarch
1 envelope unflavored gelatin
One 9-inch prepared graham cracker crumb pie crust
2 oranges, supremed (see Note)
Confectioners' sugar (optional)

In a large heavy saucepan, combine the orange juice, milk, egg yolks, sugar, cornstarch, and gelatin. Whisk until blended. Place over medium heat and cook, stirring, until the mixture is smooth and just comes to a boil. Remove from the heat, cool completely, then pour into the pie crust. Cover directly with plastic and refrigerate for at least 1 hour, or until firm.

Lay the orange sections on top of the pie in concentric circles and serve, or if you'd like to broil the orange sections, just before serving, preheat the broiler. Place the orange segments in a broiler pan and sprinkle heavily with confectioners' sugar, if using. Place 4 to 6 inches under the heat and broil until browned, watching carefully that they don't burn. Cool, then arrange the orange sections over the pie.

Makes 8 to 10 servings

Note: To supreme an orange, place the unpeeled orange on a cutting board. With a sharp paring knife, slice off the top and bottom of the orange, cutting deep enough so that no white pith remains. Sit the orange on its bottom, and working from the top downward, shave off the sides of the orange, cutting deep enough to remove all the pith. When the orange is completely peeled, cut between the membranes that divide the segments so that again no pith or membrane shows.

Recipe courtesy of the Florida Department of Citrus Headquarters

Lemon Green Tea Ice Cream

6 green tea with lemon tea bags
1¾ cups milk
2 large eggs
⅔ cup sugar
2 cups heavy cream

In a small saucepan, combine the tea bags and ½ cup of the milk. Place over medium heat and heat until bubbles are visible, then immediately take off the heat and set aside to steep for 5 minutes. Strain the tea bags, squeezing out all of the remaining liquid. In a medium bowl, beat the eggs. Temper the warm tea–milk mixture with the eggs, adding a quarter of the mixture to the beaten eggs, whisking until completely combined, then returning the mixture to the pan. Add the sugar and heavy cream and whisk vigorously until well combined. Strain into a bowl, cover, and refrigerate until cold, at least 2 hours. Transfer to an ice cream machine and churn according to the manufacturer's directions. Serve immediately or place in an airtight plastic container and freeze.

Makes 1½ quarts

Recipe courtesy of R.C. Bigelow

Butternut Squash Brûlée

4 pounds (3 to 4) butternut squash, peeled and cut into ½-inch cubes

2 pounds (about 4 medium) Russet or Yukon Gold potatoes, peeled and cut into ½-inch cubes

½ cup unsalted butter, cut into pieces and softened

1 tablespoon salt

½ teaspoon grated lime zest

1 tablespoon adobo sauce or smoked paprika, or hot pepper sauce to taste

⅔ cup packed brown sugar

Grease a 9×13×2-inch baking pan and set aside.

Place the squash and potatoes in a large pot or Dutch oven and cover with cold water. Place over medium-high heat and bring to a boil. Reduce the heat to medium-low and simmer for 10 to 15 minutes, or until soft. Drain, return to the pan, and cook over medium heat for 1 minute, stirring to evaporate excess water. Add the butter, salt, lime zest, and adobo sauce. Using an electric mixer, beat at medium speed until blended and fluffy. (The dish can be made to this point up to 1 day ahead. To reheat, bake at 350°F for 30 to 40 minutes, until heated through.)

Just before serving, preheat the broiler. Place the squash mixture in the baking pan, evenly sift the brown sugar over the top, and broil 4 to 6 inches from the heat for 5 minutes, or until the sugar bubbles and darkens slightly, watching carefully so the brown sugar doesn't burn. Remove from the oven and let cool for 5 to 10 minutes, until the brown sugar hardens. Serve immediately.

Makes 10 servings

Recipe courtesy of Andrea Laudate

SIX

※

Foods to Help You Snooze

Trouble sleeping? Before you reach for a pill, try some sleep-inducing foods. Food is without any doubt the oldest and most widely used sleeping potion, and certain foods have special powers to help you get the shut-eye you need naturally. But before we give you a rundown of those foods, be aware that adequate sleep is vital to having a healthy body, mind, and spirit.

Sleep is a time of restoration, when many important body functions occur, including tissue regeneration, muscle building, fat metabolism, and blood sugar and insulin regulation. It also provides time for learning, crystalizing memories, and solving specific problems. During the stage of sleep when dreams typically occur, the brain consolidates learned experiences and comes up with solutions to problems—hence the advice "sleep on it."

Quality sleep is also critical for recovery from mental stress. It can even make you smarter and more productive. By contrast, chronic sleep deprivation accelerates brain aging, as well as tissue degeneration and an inability to cope with day-to-day life.

When we sleep, we alternate between two types of sleep: REM (a period of rapid eye movement and dreaming) and non-REM. While you sleep, you undergo several stages of REM and non-REM sleep. Deprived of REM sleep, you're likely to lose mental focus and alertness, plus block your ability to learn new information.

Many factors can interrupt these sleep stages and compromise sleep quality:

- Sleep apnea, an obstruction of the airway, can cause you to stop breathing repeatedly during the night, forcing your brain to keep waking you up to restart your breathing. Sleep apnea can be treated successfully, and losing weight (if you are overweight) can help.

- Restless legs syndrome (RLS) can make your legs so tingly that you feel an uncontrollable urge to move them. There is a genetic component to RLS, but it can be successfully treated. Drug therapy is one option. An iron deficiency is also believed to be a culprit, so talk to your doctor about including more iron-rich foods such as lean red meats in your diet.

- Prostate problems or urinary incontinence can make you run to the bathroom several times a night.

- Medications like decongestants and high blood pressure drugs can have a stimulating effect on your brain and interfere with sleep.

- Other factors such as stress, anxiety, emotional arousal (anger, depression, excitement), caffeine, alcohol, and a disruptive environment (your sleeping area is noisy, too light, too hot, too cold, or the bed isn't comfortable) can keep you tossing and turning at night.

It's true that individual sleep patterns and sleep needs vary according to age and gender. For instance, a baby needs fourteen to fifteen hours, while an adult may need only seven to nine hours, and women tend to require more shut-eye than men do. But it's also true that with sleep in this country—like sex—no one seems to be getting enough. Nearly two thirds of Americans are suffering from sleep deprivation. Remedies abound, from sleeping pills to sleep therapy. But one solution is as close as your pantry: diet. Here's a look at some foods that can help you snooze.

Talk Turkey

That overwhelming desire to take a nap after you've enjoyed a Thanksgiving dinner comes from the turkey. Turkey contains an amino acid called tryptophan, which converts to slumber-promoting serotonin in the brain and has sedative-like properties. This chapter contains numerous turkey recipes you can incorporate into your diet in order to get a better night's sleep.

Milk It

Like turkey, milk also contains tryptophan, and calcium and magnesium in milk enhance the conversion of tryptophan to serotonin. The very best "sleeping pill" prior to bedtime just might be a turkey sandwich with a glass of milk. There's also some truth to the old wive's tale that sipping a warm beverage like milk in the evening has sleep-inducing benefits. In a study published in 1972 in the *British Medical Journal*, researchers found that a warm milk and carbohydrate drink reduced restlessness during sleep in a group of young adults and helped middle-aged adults sleep longer with fewer periods of wakefulness.

Relax with Chamomile Tea

Chamomile is considered to be a mild herbal sedative that can improve sleep quality. It contains two active compounds: angelic acid and apigenin, both of which give the herb its sedative properties. The most popular way to enjoy chamomile is as a tea. Usually you'll feel its effects within an hour. For sleep troubles, we have found that chamomile works well with other relaxation-inducing foods. After observing Gerald, a man who was suffering from insomnia, in a sleep center, we saw that his brain waves resembled a roller coaster. We treated him with a very specific diet, encouraging him to eat bananas (another tryptophan-rich food), strawberries, milk, and chamomile tea in the evening, and alertness foods such as lean proteins (eggs, fish, chicken, and lean meat) and low-carbohydrate vegetables (greens, tomatoes, broccoli, cauliflower, and so forth) for breakfast and lunch. This diet stimulated him during the day and relaxed him in the evening, for a one-two punch of good nutrition.

Chamomile tea is often an ingredient in "sleep teas," made with other herbs such as linden flower, lemon balm, lavender, and rose petals. Anyone with hay fever should avoid chamomile, however, since it is a member of the ragweed family.

Carb Up

To promote quality sleep, keep your blood sugar level on an even keel. The body considers low blood sugar a stressor and, as a result, releases the hormone cortisol, which stimulates the nervous system. Consider eating a balanced bedtime snack that includes carbohydrates. A diet rich in carbohydrates can help regulate your blood sugar and help you feel relaxed and ready for bed, because, as we've mentioned, carbs are directly involved in producing and elevating serotonin. Some carbs that may help you catch a few more winks are whole grain bread, cereals, pasta, potatoes, corn, and rice. We included a few of these in our healthy versions of comfort foods—recipes such as mashed potatoes, mac and cheese, and oatmeal. Comfort foods make you feel pleasantly relaxed and should be enjoyed from time to time.

The recipes you'll find in this chapter use these natural sleep-inducing foods to create some delicious dishes you can incorporate in your diet. They're best enjoyed in the afternoon or evening when you're ready to wind down.

SMART TIPS ● HOW TO GET MORE BRAIN BUILDING SLEEP

- Try to go to bed at a regular time each evening in order to maintain a consistent sleep schedule.

- Avoid planning for the next day. Your brain will think you're starting to work and will gear up for it, potentially keeping you awake at night. Never try to discuss heavy problems right before you go to bed.

- Relax with your breathing. Learn to focus on your breathing and nothing else.

continued

- Employ some relaxation CDs and listen to them when you want to sleep. Some resources are included in the Appendix.

- Turn off the television before going to sleep.

- Don't use cell phones, computers, or your BlackBerry just before bedtime. These gadgets in the bedroom can seriously disrupt sleeping patterns.

- Cut out sleep-robbing substances such as caffeine and alcohol.

- Avoid spicy or greasy foods as bedtime approaches. They can wreak havoc on your digestive system and keep you up at night.

- Do not do strenuous exercise at least thirty minutes before bedtime.

- If you must get up at night, try not to turn on any lights. Exposure to light in the middle of the night can block your body's production of melatonin, a hormone that regulates your sleep/wake cycle. It can make it more difficult for you to fall asleep again.

- Create a neat, restful sleep environment in your bedroom.

STARTERS AND OTHER DELIGHTS

Hot Cocoa

4 cups whole milk (or substitute lowfat milk)
½ cup unsweetened Dutch-processed cocoa powder, sifted
¼ cup superfine sugar

Place the milk in a medium heavy-duty saucepan and bring to a boil over medium heat. In a small bowl, combine the cocoa powder and sugar and toss to blend well. Add 4 tablespoons of the hot milk and stir until the mixture forms a paste. Pour the cocoa paste into the hot milk and stir until the mixture is completely smooth. Divide the hot chocolate milk among 4 mugs and serve immediately.

Makes 4 servings

Recipe courtesy of the Chocolate Council

Turkey Wings

8 turkey wings
1 teaspoon smoke essence
Salt and black pepper
Vegetable oil for frying
Smokin' Wings Hot Sauce (recipe follows)
Juice of 1 lime
2 tablespoons toasted sesame seeds
1 lime, cut into wedges, to garnish
Pickled ginger, to garnish
Wasabi paste, to garnish

Cut off the wing tips. (Reserve for turkey stock or soup.) Cut the wings into 2 pieces at each joint. In a large Dutch oven or stockpot, combine the smoke essence and salt and pepper to taste. Add the turkey wings and cold water to cover. Place over high heat and bring the wings to a boil, then immediately reduce the heat and simmer for 15 to 20 minutes, until tender. Drain and pat dry with paper towels to remove all moisture.

In a large pot, heat oil to 350 to 375°F. Deep-fry the wings, a few at a time, until they are golden brown, 6 to 8 minutes.

Remove with a slotted spoon, place the wings in a bowl, add the hot sauce and lime juice and toss gently until the wings are completely coated. Sprinkle with sesame seeds, garnish with lime wedges, pickled ginger, and wasabi paste, and serve.

Makes 4 servings (2 wings per person)

Smokin' Wings Hot Sauce

3 tablespoons Tabasco sauce
1 tablespoon sesame oil
½ cup slivered garlic
½ cup slivered ginger
½ cup finely chopped fresh cilantro

In a medium bowl, mix together the Tabasco sauce, oil, garlic, ginger, and cilantro. Cover and set aside until ready to use.

Recipe courtesy of the National Turkey Federation

Turkey Antipasto Tray

One 8-ounce package oven-roasted turkey breast slices
One 5¾-ounce can jumbo pitted black olives
One 8-ounce package turkey salami slices
One 6-ounce package provolone cheese slices
One 8-ounce package turkey ham slices
One 16-ounce jar sweet gherkins
One 6-ounce jar small sweet yellow onions
1 pound smoked turkey, cut into ½-inch cubes
One 8-ounce package turkey pastrami slices

One 3½-ounce package sesame breadsticks

1 large green bell pepper, halved and seeded

One 6-ounce jar marinated artichoke hearts

4 ounces jalapeño Monterey Jack cheese, cut into ½-inch
cubes

1 large yellow bell pepper, cut in half and seeded (optional, if
using caponata)

One 7½-ounce can caponata (optional)

Cut the oven-roasted turkey slices in 3×½-inch strips; fold the strips in half and stuff into the holes of the black olives. Alternately, layer 3 slices turkey salami with 2 slices of provolone cheese. Cut the stack into 8 wedges and spear each wedge with a toothpick. Cut the turkey ham slices in half; roll each half into a cornucopia-style horn. Place the gherkins into the center of each horn. Secure the meat and gherkin with a toothpick. On frilled toothpicks, alternately spear onions and smoked turkey cubes. Cut the turkey pastrami slices into ½-inch-wide strips. Wrap the strips around the breadsticks. Fill 1 green pepper half with marinated artichokes. Fill the other half with jalapeño Monterey Jack cheese cubes. Fill each yellow pepper half with caponata, if using.

Makes 8 to 10 servings

Recipe courtesy of the National Turkey Federation

Turkey Sausage-Stuffed Mushrooms

Nonstick cooking spray

Eight (3- to 4-inch) portobello mushrooms

1 pound hot Italian turkey sausage

1 teaspoon fennel seeds, crushed
½ cup fresh whole wheat breadcrumbs
8 ounces cream cheese, softened
⅛ teaspoon cayenne pepper
½ teaspoon salt
½ teaspoon black pepper
¼ cup olive oil
¼ cup grated Parmesan cheese

Preheat the oven to 325°F. Spray a baking sheet with nonstick cooking spray.

Remove the stems from the mushrooms and coarsely chop the stems. Squeeze the sausage from the casings into a large skillet. Place over medium heat and cook the sausage, breaking it up into small pieces. Add the chopped mushroom stems and the fennel seeds and cook until the sausage is cooked through.

Remove the mixture from the pan using a slotted spoon and place in a medium bowl. Stir in the breadcrumbs, followed by the cream cheese, cayenne, salt, and black pepper; mix well.

Place the mushroom caps on the baking sheet. Brush the mushrooms, top and bottom, with the olive oil.

Fill each mushroom cavity with ¼ cup of the sausage mixture and sprinkle with the cheese. Place in the oven and bake for 25 minutes, or until the mushrooms and stuffing are heated through.

Makes 8 servings

Recipe courtesy of the National Turkey Federation

SMART SIDE DISHES

Classic Macaroni and Cheese

2 cups dried macaroni
Nonstick cooking spray
½ cup chopped onions
½ cup nonfat evaporated milk
1 medium egg, beaten
¼ teaspoon black pepper
1¼ cups (about 4 ounces), finely shredded reduced-fat sharp
    cheddar cheese

Cook the macaroni according to the package directions. Drain and set aside. Preheat the oven to 350°F and spray a casserole dish with nonstick cooking spray.

Lightly spray a small skillet with nonstick cooking spray and place over medium heat. Add the onions and sauté for about 5 minutes, or until softened. Remove from the heat and place in a large bowl. Add the macaroni, milk, egg, pepper, and cheese and mix thoroughly. Transfer the mixture into the casserole dish and bake for 25 minutes, or until bubbly. Let stand for 10 minutes before serving.

Makes 8 servings

Source: Food Stamp Nutrition Connection

Mashed Potatoes and Celery with Yogurt

2 tablespoons kosher salt or sea salt
2½ pounds unpeeled Yukon gold potatoes, cut into ½-inch pieces

2 large celery ribs, cut into ½-inch pieces
5 cloves garlic, peeled and left whole
1 large shallot, finely chopped
2½ to 3 cups lowfat plain yogurt
Black pepper

In a large pot, bring 8 cups of water to a boil with the salt. Meanwhile, preheat the oven to 350°F. Add the potatoes, celery, and garlic to the pot. Return to a boil, then remove from heat, place in oven, and bake, uncovered, for 15 to 20 minutes, until the potatoes and celery are very tender.

Drain the potato mixture and return to the pot. Add the shallot and 2½ cups of the yogurt. With the back of a fork, mash the potatoes against sides of the pot until fairly smooth with some chunks. If you'd like the mixture creamier, add an additional ½ cup yogurt. Season with salt and pepper to taste.

Makes 8 to 10 servings

Recipe courtesy of Andrea Laudate

Pasta e Lenticchie (*Pasta with Lentils*)

1½ cups dried lentils
2½ quarts cold water
7 to 8 tablespoons olive oil
½ teaspoon red chile flakes
Salt and black pepper
1 pound dried orecchiette

Soak the lentils in a bowl of cold water for 1 hour. Discard any lentils floating on top, then drain and rinse the rest. Put the lentils with the cold water in a heatproof casserole over medium-

high heat and bring to a boil. Cover, reduce the heat, and simmer until the lentils are soft but still whole, about 45 minutes.
Drain, saving the cooking water.

Pass the lentils through a food mill, using the disc with the
smallest holes, into a medium bowl. Bring the casserole with
the cooking water back to a boil. Meanwhile, heat 5 tablespoons of the oil in a large skillet over medium heat, then add
the lentil puree, chile flakes, and salt and pepper to taste.
Sauté for 5 minutes, stirring very well to make sure the lentils
do not stick to the pan. When the cooking water reaches a
boil, add salt, and then add the pasta. Cook the pasta according to the package directions. Drain the pasta and add to the
skillet with the puréed lentils, mix very well, and cook for 30
seconds more to distribute the pasta and lentils evenly. Spoon
into bowls and serve, drizzling the remaining oil onto the
bowls.

Makes 6 servings

Recipe courtesy of Andrea Laudate

Tomato Mozzarella Bake

4 ripe beefsteak tomatoes
1 pound mozzarella cheese, grated
1 tablespoon dried basil
1 cup dried breadcrumbs

Preheat the oven to 400°F.

Halve or slice the tomatoes. (Sliced tomatoes are easier to
remove from the baking pan.) Place the tomatoes cut side up on
a baking pan with a little space between each piece. Top with

the cheese and sprinkle with the basil. Place the baking pan in the oven and, watching closely, remove the pan from the oven as soon as the cheese starts to melt and bubble. Depending on the size of your pan and number of diners, you may want to prepare a second tray for quick refills.

Makes 8 servings

Recipe courtesy of Andrea Laudate

Au Gratin Potatoes

Oil or nonstick cooking spray
6 medium (3- to 4-inch) Russet potatoes, peeled
    and ¼-inch thick
1 cup chopped onions
1½ cups shredded mild cheddar cheese
2 tablespoons margarine
4 tablespoons all-purpose flour
1 teaspoon salt
Black pepper
2 cups skim milk

Quickest Method:
Preheat the oven to 350°F.

Lightly coat a large casserole pan with oil or nonstick cooking spray.

Place a layer of potatoes in pan, using about a quarter of the potatoes. Sprinkle the layer with a quarter of the onion, cheese, margarine, flour, and salt, and a sprinkling of pepper. Repeat the layers, making a total of 4.

In a medium saucepan, heat the milk over low heat. Pour the warm milk over the mixture in the casserole dish.

Bake for 1 hour, or until potatoes are soft. Cut into serving portions and serve.

Creamiest Method:

Preheat the oven to 350°F.

Lightly coat a large casserole pan with oil or nonstick cooking spray.

Make a white sauce by melting the margarine in a small saucepan. Stir in the flour, then gradually add the milk, stirring constantly. Cook, stirring constantly, until slightly thickened. Remove from the heat. Stir in the cheese until melted and smooth. Add the salt and pepper to taste. Place a layer of potatoes and onion in the prepared casserole pan, using about a quarter of the potatoes and onions. Spread with ½ cup of the sauce. Repeat layers, making a total of 4.

Bake for 1 hour, or until potatoes are soft. Cut into serving portions and serve.

Makes 8 servings

Source: Food Stamp Nutrition Connection

BRAIN POWER ENTRÉES

Tropical Barbecue

3 tablespoons bottled barbecue sauce
1 teaspoon water

2 thin 3-ounce turkey cutlets
½ small mango, peeled, pitted, and cut into thick slices
½ medium banana, peeled and diagonally sliced
½ cup sliced button mushrooms
4 medium green onions
Nonstick cooking spray

Preheat the barbecue or a gas grill on medium. In a 9-inch pie plate, combine the barbecue sauce and water. Add the turkey and turn to coat with the sauce. Transfer the turkey to a plate and set aside. Add the remaining ingredients to the sauce and turn to coat.

Spray the rack with nonstick cooking spray. Place the turkey, fruits, and vegetables on the rack and grill for about 5 minutes, basting with the barbecue sauce and turning once, until the fruits and vegetables are browned and the turkey is no longer pink.

Makes 2 servings

Recipe courtesy of Andrea Laudate

Turkey Parmesan

⅓ cup seasoned breadcrumbs
1 pound turkey cutlets
2 to 3 teaspoons olive oil
¼ cup grated part-skim mozzarella cheese
¼ cup prepared spaghetti sauce, heated
Parmesan cheese, to serve (optional)

Place the breadcrumbs on a plate and coat the turkey thoroughly on each side with the breadcrumbs. Heat 2 teaspoons of the oil in a large nonstick skillet over medium-high heat. Add the turkey and cook for 2 to 3 minutes per side, or until the turkey is no longer pink in the center, adding the remaining teaspoon oil if needed. Sprinkle the turkey with the cheese, cover the skillet, and heat for 20 to 30 seconds, or until the cheese is melted. To serve, arrange the turkey on a platter, top with the spaghetti sauce, and finish with the Parmesan cheese, if using.

Makes 4 servings

Recipe courtesy of the National Turkey Federation

Marinated Turkey Tenderloins

½ cup white wine
1 teaspoon minced garlic
½ teaspoon dried thyme leaves
½ teaspoon salt
½ teaspoon black pepper
¼ teaspoon hot pepper sauce
1 bay leaf
2½ pounds turkey tenderloins
2 cups thinly sliced onions
Nonstick cooking spray
½ teaspoon sugar
4 slices turkey bacon, cooked and crumbled

In a large zip-top bag, combine the wine, garlic, thyme, salt, pepper, hot sauce, and bay leaf. Add the tenderloins and scatter the onions over the tenderloins. Seal the bag and refrigerate overnight.

Preheat the oven to 350°F and coat a 10×15-inch baking pan with cooking spray.

Remove the tenderloins from the marinade, reserving the marinade and onions, and place in the baking pan. Roast for 25 to 30 minutes, until the turkey is no longer pink in the center and it reaches a temperature of 160 to 165°F on a meat thermometer.

Meanwhile, in a medium nonstick skillet, combine the reserved marinade and onions. Place over medium-high heat, cook until the liquid evaporates, sprinkle with the sugar, reduce the heat to medium, and cook, stirring constantly, for 10 minutes, or until onions are golden brown.

To serve, cut each tenderloin in half. Divide the onion mixture among the tenderloins and serve topped with the crumbled bacon.

Serves 8

Recipe courtesy of the National Turkey Federation

Turkey Barbecue Meatloaf

Nonstick cooking spray
1 pound ground turkey
1 cup chopped onion
½ cup seasoned breadcrumbs
½ cup grated carrot
½ cup bottled barbecue sauce
2 teaspoons Worcestershire sauce
1 teaspoon minced garlic
¾ teaspoon black pepper

Preheat the oven and coat a 9-inch pie plate with cooking spray.

In a medium bowl, combine the turkey, onion, breadcrumbs, carrot, ¼ cup of the barbecue sauce, the Worcestershire sauce, garlic, and pepper.

Shape the mixture into a round loaf on the pie plate. Drizzle the top with the remaining ¼ cup barbecue sauce.

Bake for 35 to 45 minutes, until it reaches a temperature of 165°F when a meat thermometer is inserted in the center, the juices run clear, and the meat is no longer pink.

Makes 6 servings

Recipe courtesy of the National Turkey Federation

Turkey Breast Provençal with Vegetables

1 cup reduced-sodium turkey broth or chicken broth
¼ cup dry white wine
¼ cup fresh lemon juice
1 head garlic, cloves separated, unpeeled
One 10-ounce bag frozen whole pearl onions
2 teaspoons dried rosemary, crushed
1 teaspoon dried thyme leaves
½ teaspoon kosher salt, plus more as needed
¼ teaspoon fennel seeds, crushed
¼ teaspoon black pepper, plus more as needed
6 plum tomatoes, quartered
One 9-ounce box frozen artichoke hearts, slightly thawed
10 ounces frozen and slightly thawed or fresh asparagus spears
One 3¼-ounce can pitted black olives, drained
One 4½-pound bone-in turkey breast
Olive oil as needed

Preheat the oven to 325°F.

In a medium saucepan, combine the broth, wine, lemon juice, garlic, onions, rosemary, thyme, salt, fennel seeds, and black pepper. Cover the pan and bake for 20 minutes, or until on medium heat.

Remove the pan from the oven. Add the tomatoes, artichoke hearts, asparagus, and olives, making a pile in the center of the pan.

Rub the turkey breast with olive oil and sprinkle with salt and pepper. Place the turkey breast on top of the vegetables, breast side up. Lightly cover with foil and roast for 1 hour, basting frequently with the pan juices. Remove the foil and roast an additional 1 hour, continuing to baste, until a meat thermometer inserted in the thickest part of the breast registers 170°F.

Remove the turkey and vegetables to a serving platter. Reserve 6 cloves of garlic and the pan juices. Remove the skin from the reserved garlic. Place the garlic and pan juices in a food processor and process for 30 to 60 seconds, until the mixture is smooth. Reheat the sauce until hot. To serve, pass sauce to pour over the turkey and vegetables.

Serves 10 to 12

Recipe courtesy of the National Turkey Federation

Whole Turkey with Chestnut Turkey Sausage Stuffing

One 12-pound whole turkey (thawed if frozen)
1 teaspoon salt
1 teaspoon black pepper
1 pound turkey sausage
2 cups chopped onion

1 baguette (about 10 ounces), cut into 1-inch cubes
One 15½-ounce can chestnuts, drained
½ cup chopped fresh parsley
½ teaspoon dried thyme
½ teaspoon dried sage
1 cup reduced-sodium turkey broth or chicken broth
Red and green grapes, to garnish

Preheat the oven to 325°F.

Remove the giblets and neck from the turkey and reserve them for gravy. Rinse the turkey with cold running water and drain well. Blot dry with paper towels. Sprinkle the salt and ½ teaspoon of the pepper in the cavity of the bird. Fold the neck skin and fasten to the back with skewers. Fold the wings under the back of the turkey. Return the legs to the tucked position.

To prepare the stuffing, in large nonstick skillet, combine the turkey sausage and onions and place over medium-high heat. Cook for 5 to 7 minutes, until the sausage is no longer pink. Drain.

In a large bowl, combine the turkey sausage mixture, bread cubes, chestnuts, parsley, thyme, sage, and remaining ½ teaspoon pepper. Add the turkey broth and stir to moisten.

Lightly spoon the stuffing into the turkey or a greased 9×12-inch baking pan. (If baking separately, cover the pan and bake at 350°F for 45 minutes.)

Place the turkey, breast side up, on a rack in a large, shallow (no more than 2½ inches deep) roasting pan. Insert an oven-safe thermometer into thickest part of the thigh, taking care that it does not touch the bone. Roast the turkey for about 3½ hours, basting often with the pan juices, until the thermometer registers 180°F in the thigh, 170°F in the breast, and 165°F in the stuffing.

Remove the turkey from the oven and allow the bird to rest for 15 to 20 minutes before carving. Place on a warm large platter and garnish with the grapes.

Makes 14 servings.

Recipe courtesy of the National Turkey Federation

ENERGIZING DESSERTS

No-Bake Chocolate Peanut Butter Bars

2 cups smooth peanut butter, any type
1½ sticks unsalted butter, softened
2 cups powdered sugar
3 cups graham cracker crumbs
2 cups (one 12-ounce package) semisweet chocolate mini
   morsels

Grease a 13×9-inch baking pan and set aside.

In a large bowl, using an electric mixer, beat 1¼ cup of the peanut butter with the butter, until creamy. Gradually beat in 1 cup of the powdered sugar. With your hands or a wooden spoon, work in the remaining 1 cup powdered sugar, the graham cracker crumbs, and ½ cup of the chocolate morsels. Press the mixture evenly into the prepared baking pan and smooth the top with a spatula. Melt the remaining ¾ cup peanut butter and 1½ cups chocolate morsels in a medium, heavy-duty saucepan over the lowest possible heat, stirring constantly until smooth. Spread over the graham cracker crust in the pan. Cover and refrigerate for at least 1 hour, or until the chocolate is firm, then cut into bars. Store in the refrigerator.

Makes 12 servings

Recipe courtesy of Andrea Laudate

Old-Fashioned Bread Pudding

5 slices white or whole wheat bread
2 tablespoons margarine or unsalted butter
¼ teaspoon ground cinnamon
⅓ cup white or brown sugar
½ cup raisins
3 large eggs or 1 large egg plus 2 egg whites
1½ cups skim milk, if using microwave, or 2 cups if using oven
¼ teaspoon salt
1 teaspoon vanilla extract

Spread one side of each slice of bread with butter. Sprinkle with the cinnamon. Cut into 1-inch cubes. In a lightly sprayed casserole dish, combine the bread, sugar, and raisins.

Microwave method: In a medium bowl, whisk together the eggs, 1½ cups milk, salt, and vanilla. Pour over the bread mixture and gently combine. Cover, microwave on high for 5 minutes, then turn the dish a quarter turn. Microwave on high for 3 to 5 minutes longer, until the edges are firm and the center is almost set. Let sit, covered, for 10 minutes before serving. Serve warm or chilled.

Oven method: Preheat the oven to 350°F. In a medium bowl, whisk together the eggs, 2 cups milk, the salt, and vanilla. Pour over the bread mixture and gently combine. Place in the oven and bake, uncovered, for 1 hour, or until a knife inserted in the pudding comes out clean. Serve warm or cold.

Makes 6 servings

Source: Food Stamp Nutrition Connection

Indian Pudding

2½ cups skim milk
½ cup skim milk, chilled
½ cup cornmeal
1 tablespoon margarine
¼ to ½ cup molasses
½ teaspoon ground ginger
½ teaspoon ground cinnamon

Preheat the oven to 325°F. Lightly grease a 1-quart baking pan.

In a medium saucepan, heat the 2½ cups milk over medium heat to reach a simmer. In a small bowl, mix together the ½ cup cold milk with the cornmeal. Add the cornmeal mixture to warm milk and stir well. Cook for 20 minutes over medium-low heat until thickened, stirring often to prevent scorching. Remove the pudding from the heat. Stir in the margarine, molasses, ginger, and cinnamon. Pour into the baking pan and bake for 55 to 60 minutes, until a knife inserted in the center comes out clean. Cool slightly, then cut into 8 squares and serve warm.

Makes 8 servings

Source: Food Stamp Nutrition Connection

Pineapple Rice Bake

Nonstick cooking spray or oil
4 large eggs
1 cup milk
½ cup sugar
One 8-ounce can crushed pineapple, undrained
½ teaspoon ground cinnamon (optional)
½ teaspoon ground nutmeg (optional)
1 teaspoon vanilla extract
3 cups cooked rice

Preheat the oven to 350°F. Lightly coat an ovenproof 2-quart casserole dish with cooking spray or oil.

In a large bowl, beat together the eggs, milk, and sugar. Add the pineapple, cinnamon, nutmeg, and vanilla. Stir in the rice. Pour into the casserole dish and bake for 50 to 60 minutes, until a knife inserted in the center of the pudding comes out clean. Serve in custard dishes.

Makes 6 servings

Source: Food Stamp Nutrition Connection

SEVEN

❀

Good Mood Foods

When we're feeling down in the dumps, we often instinctively turn to food to cheer us up or lift our spirits. And believe it or not, we're on the right track: For more than forty years, scientists have known that food alters our brain chemistry in ways that profoundly influence our moods. In fact, poor diet quality, ubiquitous in the United States, is now considered a modifiable risk factor for depression. Diet can have definite behavioral effects.

The problem, though, is that many of the foods we reach for when we're depressed will lift our spirits momentarily but later make them crash. Those "comfort foods" include indulgences like ice cream, milk and cookies, and chips—foods that are laced with sugar, fat, and salt. While they may temporarily deflate a blue mood, they ultimately will inflate your waistline—and only make the bad days worse.

The encouraging news is that not all comfort foods are

unhealthful for you. There are plenty of effective mood-lifting foods to choose from. Remarkably, you can manipulate your brain chemistry to stay upbeat simply by what you put on your plate and by indulging in foods that induce a natural, healthy high. Most of these foods are common, everyday staples. Here's a rundown.

Go for the Green

Popeye the Sailor downed spinach for strength; now you can eat it for mental vigor. Spinach and other green leafy vegetables are loaded with folic acid, a member of the B vitamin family. Folic acid does a number of good deeds in the body, one of which is maintaining healthy levels of serotonin. Additionally, it is one of three B vitamins that reduce the brain- and heart-damaging protein homocysteine in the body. Others are vitamin B_6 and vitamin B_{12}. Homocysteine technically is an amino acid, and when it piles up in the body, damage to the inner walls of the arteries can ensue. Some scientists theorize that, in addition to increasing one's risk of stroke by gumming up carotid arteries that carry oxygen to the brain, high homocysteine levels can cause a neurotransmitter deficiency, which leads to a depressed mood. To ensure that you get enough folic acid, eat not only dark green leafy vegetables such as spinach and romaine lettuce, but also legumes and beans, cauliflower, lean meats, eggs, and nuts.

Fish for a Good Mood

Fish is not only brain food; it's mood food. A growing body of research is showing that consuming fish can reduce the symptoms of depression.

Why is fish such a mood elevator? The answer is that it is rich in omega-3 fatty acids. One of these is an omega-3 fat known as docosahexaenoic acid (DHA). About one third of the fat in your brain is DHA. Considered a building block of the brain, DHA is required for normal brain and eye development, as well as for mental well-being and functioning. Your brain loves DHA; it takes up this fat in preference to other fatty acids.

Low levels of DHA are linked to depression. A study published in the medical journal *Lancet* stated that in regions where people eat more fish, there are fewer cases of depression. And according to a report in the *American Journal of Clinical Nutrition*, the documented increase in poor nutrition in North America over the last century parallels the dwindling consumption of DHA over the same period. In other research, scientists have examined the cell membranes of people suffering from depression to assess cellular DHA levels. One study of fifteen depressed patients and fifteen healthy volunteers found that depressed patients had significant depletions of fatty acids, particularly DHA, in the cell membranes of their red blood cells. There's clearly a connection between depression and levels of DHA in the body.

Exactly how DHA and other omega-3 fats help alleviate depression is still a question mark. But there are some clues. Some research indicates that higher levels of these fats in the body may lead to increased levels of neurotransmitters, particularly serotonin, the chemical most responsible for boosting mood.

To take advantage of DHA's power, enjoy fish a few times a week. Good choices include salmon, tuna, sardines, snapper, oysters, and many other species of fish and shellfish. Walnuts are also high in omega-3 fats.

Discover Brazil Nuts

These tasty nuts are filled with selenium, an antioxidant mineral with a windfall of benefits. Widely recognized as a cancer preventative, this mineral is also finding favor as a mood elevator because it is important to the functioning of the brain. The metabolism of selenium by the brain differs from other organs. When selenium is in short supply, the brain retains it to a greater extent than other nutrients. This preferential retention of selenium in the brain suggests that it is important to our brain power. Bolstering that suggestion, numerous studies report that a low selenium intake is associated with poorer mood. Bottom line: The brain loves selenium.

We recommend that you get your selenium naturally from food, and Brazil nuts are one of the best sources. Grown in selenium-rich soil, a single nut supplies nearly twice the recommended daily amount of selenium (55 micrograms). If you think you're getting less than the recommended amount, introduce more lean meat, chicken, organ meats, seafood, and whole grains into your diet. If you don't have Brazil nuts lying around, you can meet your entire daily selenium requirement in another way: by eating a tuna salad sandwich on whole wheat bread for lunch. If you're already taking a multivitamin that contains selenium, don't take a selenium supplement; the mineral can be toxic in very high amounts.

Soothe with Milk

The calcium in milk and other dairy products can make you feel less irritable or depressed, with fewer mood swings, and it can subdue menstrual blues. The reason for calcium's amazing powers has to do with the mineral's role in maintaining normal nerve function. Milk and other dairy products are a blend of protein and natural sugars—a combination that helps stabilize blood sugar for a more even mood. The body hates low blood sugar because the brain needs a constant blood sugar level to function optimally. Your best sources of mood-mellowing calcium are milk, yogurt, and cottage cheese. If you're lactose intolerant or dislike dairy products, turn to calcium-rich vegetables such as broccoli, dark greens such as kale, or turnip greens.

Zone Out on a Little Chocolate

That Valentine's Day candy you enjoy every February, or the sweet stuff you munch on in the movie theater, are actually a conglomeration of natural chemicals that have a near-narcotic effect on your mood. One is theobromine, a stimulant similar to caffeine that perks you up. Another is phenylethylamine (PEA), which makes you feel lovey-dovey toward a person to whom you're attracted. There's also a substance in chocolate called anandamide that interacts with brain cells in much the same matter as marijuana. You can't get high on chocolate, though, unless you eat about a quarter of your weight in chocolate in a single sitting. Last but not least, chocolate candy contains sugar, which produces a temporary energy and serotonin boost. Chocolate, in all its incarnations, is a bona fide picker-upper, and should be enjoyed in delightful moderation.

OTHER MOOD-BOOSTING FOODS

Barley
Beans
Brown rice
Bulgur wheat
Chocolate
Corn
Garlic
Greens
Legumes
Oats
Potatoes
Pumpkin
Squash
Sweet potatoes
Turnips
Wild rice
Yams

SMART TIPS ● MORE WAYS TO BOOST YOUR MOOD

- **SEEK THERAPY.** Counseling can help you identify why your depression exists and give you constructive guidelines for resolving it. Consider cognitive therapy. It can teach you how to slip out of self-defeating thought patterns and think more positively and realistically about the world around you.

- **GET MOVING.** Exercise is emerging as an important adjunct to counseling. One reason is that it releases natural mood-elevating

continued

chemicals called endorphins. Try walking or dancing for reducing depression.

- **MODIFY YOUR ENVIRONMENT.** Moods can worsen if you're lonely or isolated—or in surroundings or around people who bring you down. You may have to change your lifestyle, make new contacts, or consider volunteering for a good cause.

- **LOOK FOR INSPIRATION.** Begin reading inspirational books or material that will uplift you and help you to feel more hopeful.

- **LAUGH OFTEN AND MUCH.** Laughter has often been called the tranquilizer with no side effects. And for good reason. It stimulates the pituitary gland in your brain, in turn releasing endorphins for a natural high. When you laugh, you automatically draw in a deep breath. This expands your lungs and increases blood and oxygen circulation, in much the same way deep breathing or exercise does. The net effect is relaxation and mood elevation.

- **HAVE A PHYSICAL CHECKUP.** There are many conditions that produce depressive symptoms, including thyroid malfunction, menopause, diabetes, and anemia. See your doctor to rule out medical reasons for the blues.

STARTERS AND OTHER DELIGHTS

Chocolate Shake

1 cup lowfat milk
1 scoop fat-free chocolate ice cream
Chopped pecans or walnuts, to garnish

Place the milk and ice cream in the blender. Blend until smooth, then pour into a glass and garnish with chopped nuts. Serve immediately.

Makes 1 large serving

Recipe courtesy of Maggie Greenwood-Robinson

Texas Lentil Dip

1 cup dried lentils, washed and drained
2 cups water
¼ cup mayonnaise
¼ cup sour cream
1 teaspoon dry mustard
1 teaspoon red pepper flakes
Salt
Tortilla chips, to serve

Combine the lentils and water in a medium saucepan. Place over medium-high heat, bring to a boil, then reduce the heat, cover, and simmer for 40 minutes, or until soft. Drain and mash the lentils in a large bowl. Add the remaining ingredients with salt to taste and mix well. Serve with tortilla chips.

Makes 6 servings

Recipe courtesy of the USA Dry Pea and Lentil Council

Sardine Spread

Two 3¾-ounce cans sardines
¼ cup fresh lemon juice

½ teaspoon hot pepper sauce
½ cup bottled chili sauce

Drain the sardines and place in a medium bowl. Mash the sardines and add the lemon juice, hot pepper sauce, and chili sauce. Spread on bread or toast for a quick high-protein sandwich or serve on crackers for a snack.

Yields about 1½ cups

Recipe courtesy of Bumble Bee

Tuna Appetizer

One 8-ounce package cream cheese, softened
One 16-ounce jar prepared salsa
One 12-ounce can solid white tuna, drained and flaked
1 green onion, sliced
2 ounces (½ cup) shredded cheddar cheese
One 10-ounce bag tortilla chips

Spread the softened cream cheese in a 9-inch microwave-safe pie plate. Top with the salsa, then the tuna. Sprinkle with the green onion and cheese. Microwave on high for 4 minutes or chill and serve cold. Serve with tortilla chips.

Makes about 2 cups

Recipe courtesy of Bumble Bee

Fiesta Mix

1 cup cereal with fruit bits, any brand
1 cup Chex cereal

1 cup O-shaped cereal
¼ cup raisins
¼ cup peanuts
¼ cup shredded unsweetened coconut flakes

In a large bowl, mix the cereals together. Add the raisins, peanuts, and coconut; mix well.

Makes 4 servings

Source: Food Stamp Nutrition Connection

SMART SIDE DISHES

Corn Sticks

Nonstick cooking spray or all-purpose flour
1¼ cups white or yellow cornmeal
⅔ cup all-purpose flour
2 to 4 tablespoons sugar (you'll need less if white cornmeal is used)
1 tablespoon baking powder
½ teaspoon salt
1 large egg, beaten
1 cup milk
¼ cup vegetable oil
3 tablespoons mayonnaise

Preheat the oven to 375°F. Spray 14 corn stick molds with cooking spray and coat with flour. Place molds in the oven while it preheats, about 15 minutes.

In a large bowl, combine the cornmeal, flour, sugar, baking powder, and salt. Add the egg, milk, oil, and mayonnaise to the dry ingredients and mix well. Remove molds from the oven and pour the batter into molds. Bake at 375° for 10 to 15 minutes, or until golden brown or until a toothpick inserted in the center of corn stick comes out clean. Cool in molds on wire racks for 10 minutes. Remove corn sticks from molds; serve warm.

Makes 14 corn sticks

Kale and Parsnips

1 tablespoon corn oil
1 cup halved and sliced onions
1 cup halved and sliced parsnips
1 cup water
2 tablespoons minced ginger
1 bunch kale, stalks removed, and cut into bite-size pieces

Heat the oil in a large sauté pan over medium heat. Add the onions and parsnips and sauté for 5 minutes, stirring occasionally to prevent burning. Add the water and ginger, cover, and simmer for 4 to 5 minutes, until the vegetables are tender. Add the kale and cook 4 to 5 minutes longer, stirring occasionally, until softened. Serve hot.

Makes 4 servings

Recipe courtesy of the Pioneer Valley Growers Association

Summer Salad

Two 16-ounce cans black beans, drained and rinsed
Two 16-ounce cans chickpeas, drained and rinsed
1 cup cooked yellow corn kernels
3 large tomatoes, chopped
1 Vidalia onion, diced
1 large red bell pepper, chopped
¾ cup red wine vinegar
2 tablespoons finely chopped fresh cilantro, or more to taste
2 tablespoons fresh lime juice
Salt and black pepper

In a large bowl, combine all the ingredients, with salt and pepper to taste. Mix well, cover, and refrigerate for 4 hours before serving. Mix the salad again before serving.

Makes 10 servings

Recipe courtesy of the Georgia Fruit and Vegetable Growers Association

Marinated Slaw

4 cups chopped green cabbage
½ cup chopped red cabbage
1 teaspoon grated lemon zest
4 tablespoons chopped cucumber
5 tablespoons chopped carrot
1 tablespoon chopped red bell pepper
1 tablespoon chopped green bell pepper
6 tablespoons chopped Vidalia onion
2 tablespoons grated radish

3 hard-cooked egg whites, chopped
½ teaspoon salt
½ teaspoon black pepper
½ teaspoon dried oregano
1 teaspoon sugar
1 teaspoon apple cider vinegar
4 tablespoons mayonnaise
5 tablespoons bottled Italian dressing

In a large bowl, combine the cabbage, lemon zest, cucumber, carrot, bell peppers, onion, radish, and egg whites, mixing well. In a small bowl, combine the salt, pepper, oregano, and sugar. Add to the cabbage mixture and toss until well blended. In a small bowl, whisk together the vinegar, mayonnaise, and Italian dressing. Pour over the slaw, tossing until thoroughly coated. Cover and chill overnight.

Makes 10 servings

Recipe courtesy of the Georgia Fruit and Vegetable Growers Association

Spinach-Corn Salsa

Two 15-ounce cans spinach, drained
One 15-ounce can whole kernel corn
One 15-ounce can whole tomatoes with juice
1 small white or red onion, diced
1 or 2 medium to large fresh tomatoes, diced
3 cloves garlic, diced
4 sprigs of cilantro, diced
Several splashes of balsamic vinegar or red wine vinegar
1 to 2 dashes cayenne pepper or 1 jalapeño chile, diced

In a large bowl, mix all the ingredients together, crushing the tomatoes as you mix. Serve at room temperature, or refrigerate and serve cold. Serve as a salsa with chips or as a vegetable side dish.

Makes 6 servings

Source: U.S. Department of Health and Human Services, Indian Health,
Division of Diabetes Treatment and Prevention

BRAIN POWER ENTRÉES

Bow-Tie Tuna Salad

4 ounces cooked bow-tie pasta
1 cup red and green seedless grapes, halved
One 3-ounce can tuna, drained and flaked
½ cup coarsely chopped walnuts
¼ cup lowfat lemon yogurt
Lettuce leaves, to serve

Place the bow ties in a medium bowl. Add the grapes, tuna, and walnuts. Stir in the yogurt, mixing well. Arrange lettuce leaves on 2 or 3 plates. Spoon the salad onto the lettuce, dividing evenly among the plates. (If you like, you can chill up to 6 hours before serving.)

Makes 2 to 3 servings

Recipe courtesy of Bumble Bee

Easy Walnut Fettuccine Alfredo

1 cup walnut pieces

½ cup water

1 cup skim milk

1 tablespoon all-purpose flour

1 clove garlic, minced

½ teaspoon kosher salt or ¼ teaspoon table salt

¼ teaspoon black pepper

8 ounces uncooked fettuccine noodles

1½ cups frozen petits pois

¾ cup (about 3 ounces) shredded Parmesan cheese

1 ounce prosciutto, cut into thin strips

Place the walnuts and water in a food processor. Process until very smooth and set aside.

In a medium saucepan, whisk together the milk and flour. Place over medium heat; add the garlic, salt, and pepper; and bring to a simmer. Simmer, stirring, until slightly thickened and smooth, about 3 minutes. Stir in the walnut mixture and cook, stirring, over low heat until thickened, 1 to 2 minutes.

Meanwhile, cook the pasta according to the package directions, adding the peas during the last 2 minutes of cooking time. Drain.

Add the pasta, peas, and cheese to the sauce. Cook, stirring, over low heat until just heated through and the pasta is evenly coated with sauce. Top each serving with a few strips of prosciutto.

Makes 6 servings

Recipe courtesy of the Walnut Marketing Board

Walnut Veggie Tacos

One 14-ounce can diced tomatoes with juice or 1½ cups
   chopped fresh tomatoes
2 cups (about 2 medium) diced zucchini
2 tablespoons taco seasoning mix (half of a 1.35-ounce packet)
2 tablespoons water
One 14-ounce can black beans, rinsed and drained
¾ cup frozen or drained canned corn kernels
¾ cup chopped walnuts
6 taco shells or 6-inch flour or corn tortillas
Shredded lettuce, shredded cheese, sour cream, and avocado
   slices, to serve

In a wide skillet, combine the tomatoes and zucchini. Place
over medium heat, bring to a simmer, and cook, uncovered, for
3 minutes, or until zucchini is soft. Stir in the taco seasoning,
water, black beans, and corn. Bring to a simmer, cover, and
simmer for 5 minutes. Stir in the walnuts, remove from the
heat, and let stand for 1 to 2 minutes for the sauce to thicken.
Serve in the taco shells or tortillas with your choice of condiments.

Makes 6 servings

Recipe courtesy of the Walnut Marketing Board

Bar-B-Q Lentils

2⅓ cups dried lentils, rinsed
5 cups water
½ cup molasses
2 tablespoons brown sugar

1 tablespoon apple cider vinegar
½ cup ketchup
1 teaspoon dry mustard
1 teaspoon Worcestershire sauce
One 16-ounce can tomato sauce
2 tablespoons minced onion
¼ teaspoon liquid smoke (optional)

Preheat the oven to 350°F.

In a large ovenproof saucepan, combine the lentils with the water. Place over medium-high heat and bring to a boil. Reduce the heat and simmer for 30 minutes, or until the lentils are tender but still whole. Add the remaining ingredients and stir to combine. Place the pan in the oven and bake for 45 minutes.

Makes 8 servings

Recipe courtesy of the USA Dry Pea and Lentil Council

Apple-Tuna Sandwiches

1 apple
One 6½-ounce can drained water-packed tuna
¼ cup lowfat vanilla yogurt
1 teaspoon prepared mustard
1 teaspoon honey
6 slices whole wheat bread
3 lettuce leaves

Peel and core the apple and chop into small pieces. In a medium bowl, combine the tuna, apple, yogurt, mustard, and honey. Stir well. Spread ½ cup of the tuna mixture onto each of 3 slices of bread. Top each sandwich with a lettuce leaf and the remaining bread slices.

Makes 3 servings

Source: Food Stamp Nutrition Connection

ENERGIZING DESSERTS

Chocolate Sorbet

1¼ cups water
¾ cup superfine sugar
⅓ cup unsweetened Dutch-processed cocoa powder, sifted
4 ounces bittersweet or semisweet chocolate, finely chopped

In a 2-quart saucepan, combine the water and sugar. Place over medium heat and bring to a boil, stirring to dissolve the sugar. Add the cocoa powder and stir until it is dissolved and the mixture is smooth. Remove the pan from the heat and add the chopped chocolate. Stir until completely melted. Strain the mixture into a bowl. Cover tightly with plastic wrap and cool to room temperature, then refrigerate for several hours or overnight to completely chill. Process in an ice cream maker according to the manufacturer's instructions.

Makes 1 pint

Recipe courtesy of the Chocolate Council

Xtreme Chocolate Frappe

⅓ cup sugar
2 tablespoons cocoa powder
2 cups lowfat milk
¼ cup light chocolate syrup
1 teaspoon vanilla extract
Two 6-ounce containers lowfat chocolate, vanilla, or plain
    yogurt
4 ice cubes
Bittersweet chocolate shavings, to serve (optional)

In a small saucepan, mix together the sugar and cocoa powder. Add ½ cup of the milk and place over medium-low heat. Cook, stirring constantly, for 3 minutes, or until the mixture is hot and the sugar is dissolved. Pour the mixture into a blender.

Add the remaining 1½ cups milk, the chocolate syrup, vanilla, yogurt, and ice cubes to the blender and blend until smooth. Pour into 6 glasses and sprinkle with chocolate shavings or additional cocoa powder.

Makes 6 servings

Recipe courtesy of Dairy Management Inc.

Chocolate-Dipped Fruit and Nuts

1 pound bittersweet or white chocolate

FRUIT
Large or long-stemmed fresh strawberries
Fresh or dried pear slices
Fresh or dried apple slices

Dried pineapple slices
Dried pear slices
Dried apricot halves
Dried banana chips
Dried peaches
Dried plums

NUTS
Cashews
Brazil nuts
Walnuts
Almonds
Pecans
Hazelnuts
Macadamia nuts

Line 2 baking sheets with parchment or wax paper.

Melt and temper the chocolate: Chop the chocolate into very small pieces and set aside a third of it. Melt the remaining two thirds in the top of a double boiler over hot, not simmering, water, stirring frequently with a rubber spatula to ensure even melting. The chocolate should not exceed 120°F (110°F for white chocolate). Remove the top of the double boiler and wipe it dry. Stir in the remaining chocolate in three batches, making sure that each batch is completely melted before adding the next. When all the chocolate has been added, test the chocolate by dipping your finger in and placing a dab of chocolate just below your lower lip. If it is comfortable, not too hot or too cool, the temperature is correct. If the chocolate is too warm, stir in more finely chopped chocolate, or continue to stir and test again until the chocolate is tempered. If the temperature of the finished chocolate is lower than it should be, warm the chocolate over hot water just until it reaches the correct temperature.

Hold the fruit and larger nuts securely between your thumb and forefinger and dip them into the chocolate, covering by three quarters.

Remove from the chocolate, gently shake off the excess, and place on the prepared pan. Repeat with the remaining fruits and nuts. Let the chocolate set at room temperature or chill in the refrigerator for 15 minutes.

The dipped fresh fruits must be served within 4 hours of preparation; if you're not serving immediately, refrigerate until 15 minutes before serving. Makes 1 pound of bittersweet or white chocolate, finely chopped and tempered.

Recipe courtesy of the Chocolate Council

Cocoa Angel Food Cake

1 cup all-purpose flour, sifted
3 tablespoons unsweetened cocoa powder, sifted
1½ cups superfine sugar
¼ teaspoon salt
12 large egg whites, at room temperature
1 teaspoon cream of tartar
1 tablespoon vanilla extract

Position a rack in the center of the oven and preheat the oven to 325°F.

In a medium bowl, thoroughly combine the flour, cocoa powder, ¾ cup of the superfine sugar, and the salt. Set aside. Place the remaining ¾ cup superfine sugar in a measuring cup near the mixer.

In the grease-free bowl of an electric stand mixer using the wire whip, or in a mixing bowl using a handheld mixer, beat the egg whites on low speed until slightly frothy. Add the cream of tartar and whip the egg whites until they begin to form peaks. Raise the speed to medium and slowly sprinkle on the remaining ¾ cup superfine sugar, about 2 tablespoons at a time, then continue whipping the whites until firm but not dry. Blend in the vanilla, then remove the bowl from the mixer.

Sprinkle the dry ingredients over the whipped egg whites, about 3 tablespoons at a time, and gently fold them into the whites using a long-handled rubber spatula.

Turn the batter into a 10×4-inch tube pan, preferably with a removable bottom. Use the rubber spatula to smooth and even the top. Tap the pan on the countertop gently a few times to eliminate any air bubbles.

Place the cake in the oven and bake until it is golden brown, it springs back when lightly touched, and a cake tester inserted near the center comes out clean, about 40 minutes. Remove the pan from the oven and immediately invert it onto its feet, or hang it by the center tube over a funnel or the neck of a bottle. Leave the cake to hang for several hours, until completely cooled.

To remove the cake from the pan, run a thin-bladed knife, preferably serrated, around the inside of the pan and around the tube using a sawing motion. Gently loosen the cake from the edges and push the bottom of the pan up, away from the sides. Run the knife between the bottom of the cake and the bottom of the pan and invert the cake onto a plate, then reinvert so it is right side up.

The cake will keep at room temperature, well wrapped in plastic, for 3 days, or it can be frozen for up to 3 weeks. If frozen, defrost in the refrigerator for 24 hours before serving.

Makes 14 to 16 servings

Recipe courtesy of the Chocolate Council

Fruit Pizza

COOKIE CRUST

½ cup margarine

½ cup sugar

1 teaspoon vanilla extract

1 large egg

2 cups all-purpose flour

2 teaspoons baking powder

CHEESE SPREAD

8 ounces reduced-fat or fat-free cream cheese, softened

½ cup sugar

1 teaspoon vanilla extract

FRUIT TOPPINGS

1 cup sliced strawberries, kiwis, bananas, pears, peaches, or blueberries

Preheat the oven to 375°F.

To make the cookie crust, in a medium bowl, cream together the margarine, sugar, vanilla, and egg until light and fluffy. Add the flour and baking powder and mix well. Spread the mixture about ⅛ inch thick on a pizza pan, baking sheet, or 9 × 13 × 2-inch baking pan. Place in the oven and bake for 10 to 12 minutes, until lightly browned. Remove from the oven and cool on a wire rack. To make the cheese spread, in a medium bowl, cream together the cream cheese, sugar, and vanilla. Spread over the cooled cookie crust. Arrange the fruit on top of the pizza. Refrigerate until ready to serve.

Makes 12 servings

Source: Food Stamp Nutrition Connection

EIGHT

※

Edging Out Anger

Anger is not always the result of an incident, like a car pulling out in front of you on the highway, or your spouse bouncing a check, or losing that big promotion. It can stem from something in your diet, like a nutrient deficiency or low blood sugar. In psychological circles, an outburst caused by a nutritional debt is termed a "hot brain," meaning that the brain overreacts to something in the environment (a stimulus). A nutritional debt can also lead to lack of inhibition. This means someone might act more spontaneously, or unpredictably, than the average person, or they might not have control over their responses. Children, for example, might start using vulgar language as a result of lack of inhibition. But as soon as they regain nutritional strength, they use more polite and courteous behavior because they can better think through and anticipate the consequences of their behavior. We've seen this happen.

But let us say this: Anger is not necessarily a bad thing. It can serve a useful purpose by making you realize something is wrong and needs to be fixed. It can prime you to action. Even so, it's important to vent your anger appropriately, and not stay mad, since unresolved anger can significantly affect your health and well-being. Anger turned inward (unvented) increases stress and anxiety and leads to depression, for example. So don't wallow in your misery. Try to do something else such as a project that diverts your attention away from the object of your anger. If you feel tense and irritable, relax by listening to soothing music. Move your body, too. Increasing your physical activity can clear away feelings of anger and irritability.

Equally important is putting the right fuel in your body. In fact, research is revealing more and more specific benefits from certain foods when it comes to quelling anger and irritable moods. If you're a woman, you're aware probably that upping the amount of complex carbohydrates you eat, such as whole grains and beans, can help relieve many symptoms of PMS, including tension and anger. That's because carbs swell the ranks of the feel-good chemical serotonin in your body. But that's only the beginning of "nutritional anger management techniques" that come straight from your kitchen. Take a look.

Eat More Often

Shoot for five or six mini-meals, instead of three squares a day, if you're anger-prone or feel on the edge. This habit will help you maintain a steady blood sugar level and prevent irritability. Plan your meals with a good balance of complex carbohydrates and a moderate amount of protein (a small tuna sandwich on whole grain bread, for example). This style of eating can help mellow you out if you tend to fly off the handle.

Wean Yourself Off High Stimulants, Such as Caffeine

Beverages containing caffeine, including coffee, tea, and soft drinks, can increase anxiety, irritability, and mood swings in adults. If you're a victim of any of these mood states, you'll want to start cutting back gradually (withdrawal can induce head-aches and may take a week) by substituting decaffeinated coffee, grain-based coffee substitutes, and caffeine-free herbal teas. You may also have a low-grade allergy to these stimulants, which results in toxicity in the brain.

Go Complex (Carbohydrates, That Is)

As we mentioned above, carbohydrates are the dietary building blocks of serotonin, but not all carbs are equally good at building serotonin. Simple carbohydrates such as sugar, syrup, or honey will boost your blood sugar and serotonin levels only temporarily. After an initial high or feeling of calm, you may feel irritable or moody again. You'll want to choose complex carbohydrates instead to keep your anger and irritability under wraps. A good example of how well this works is Rosita, a very angry and frustrated mother. Not coincidentally, she was addicted to sugar and constantly munched on candy bars and hard candy. Among the tools we offered her to help manage her angry disposition was a nutritional plan. Part of it involved not eating any sugar for thirty days to detox her body, as would happen in any addiction program. A mainstay of her new diet was wholesome, high-fiber complex carbohydrates such as fruit and whole grains. She began to feel better very quickly, and her volatility diminished greatly.

As Rosita did, try easing back on simple sugars and add the following complex carbohydrates to your shopping list: whole grains, beans and legumes, seeds and nuts, vegetables, and fresh fruits. Complex carbs are also high in a variety of B vitamins. When these nutrients are in short supply, one of the first signs of deficiency is irritability and fatigue.

Keep Your Calcium and Magnesium in Balance

The minerals calcium and magnesium work together to transmit messages throughout your nervous system. Calcium temporarily increases the release of stress hormones such as adrenaline, while magnesium suppresses excess adrenaline. Many women, in particular, take in a great deal of calcium through food and supplements, which may tilt them toward a relative magnesium deficiency, creating feelings of nervousness and irritability. It's not necessary that you cut back on your calcium intake, but make sure your diet is magnesium rich. Some good sources include fish, seeds, avocado, beans, whole grains, and dark green vegetables. And if you take a calcium supplement, take magnesium as well.

Feel Good on Fish

Docosahexaenoic acid (DHA), one of the healthy omega-3 fats in fish, can reduce aggressive and hostile behavior, including aggressive driving, bullying, verbal abusiveness, and fighting. Several studies have found that omega-3 and nutrient status tends to be impaired in criminals, and that supplementation consisting of 100 percent of the requirement for vitamins, minerals, and essential fatty acids could reduce the incidence of insubordination among inmates. That's fairly compelling proof that good nutrition can work wonders on problem behavior. As we've stated throughout this book, fish and its wealth of omega-3 fats are vital for optimum brain health. Mounds of scientific evidence reveal that omega-3 fats combat depression, improve intellectual performance, rebuild the fatty membranes of brain cells, and protect against stroke. The current recommendation for optimum physical and mental health is to eat two to three fish meals a week.

Get in the Zinc Sync

Zinc is at the heart of many activities in your body. For example, it helps absorb vitamins; break down carbohydrates; synthesize nucleic acid, which directs the manufacture of protein in cells; and regulate the growth and development of reproductive organs. Zinc is also a component of insulin, and it prevents deficiencies that can lead to problems in your body's use of insulin, including low blood sugar.

Once in the bloodstream, zinc levels are regulated by a metal-binding protein called metallothionein. In many people with angry or disordered behavior, this protein malfunctions, creating a zinc deficiency. When zinc levels are restored through diet or supplementation, behavior often improves.

Zinc-poor diets are also associated with cardiovascular disease, high blood pressure, elevated triglycerides, and impaired glucose tolerance. Foods high in zinc include meats, oysters and other shellfish, poultry, potatoes, lima beans, whole grains, peas, and milk.

Pretty amazing, isn't it, that proper nutrition is one tool you can use to help you cope? Of course, if your irritability is severe and unrelenting, you'll want to talk to your doctor or be referred to a psychologist. But at the very least, a healthier diet will help your mood because you'll have more energy to deal with whatever is triggering your anger. What follows is a list of recipes that can help you get started on a path to calm.

SMART TIPS ● ANGER MANAGEMENT

- Imagine the source of your anger as a balloon, and see it floating away until it is no longer in your mind's eye.

- Read inspirational books or passages on the power of forgiveness.

- Try aggressive exercises such as boxing or beating your bed with a tennis racket to vent your anger.

- Journal your feelings and fears in a diary to allow your mind to expel your negative emotions.

- Learn to recognize when your anger is building, and then develop an imaginary inner off-switch to turn it down.

- In a situation that triggers anger, take several deep breaths or remove yourself from the situation.

STARTERS AND OTHER DELIGHTS

Blackberry Smoothie

1 cup milk, chilled
½ cup fresh or frozen blackberries or raspberries
1 to 3 tablespoons sugar, to taste
½ cup crushed ice

Place all the ingredients in a blender and blend until smooth.
Pour into a glass and serve immediately.

Makes 1 serving

Recipe courtesy of the North American Bramble Growers Association

Blackberry Breakfast Bars

2 cups fresh or frozen blackberries or raspberries
2 tablespoons sugar
2 tablespoons water
1 tablespoon fresh lemon juice
¾ teaspoon ground cinnamon
1 cup all-purpose flour
1 cup quick-cooking rolled oats
⅔ cup packed brown sugar
⅛ teaspoon baking soda
½ cup margarine or unsalted butter, melted

Preheat the oven to 350°F.

To make the filling, in a medium saucepan, combine the berries, sugar, water, lemon juice, and ½ teaspoon of the cinnamon. Place over medium heat and bring to a boil. Reduce the heat and simmer, uncovered, for about 8 minutes, or until slightly thickened, stirring frequently. Remove from the heat.

In a medium bowl, stir together the flour, oats, brown sugar, remaining ¼ teaspoon cinnamon, and the baking soda. Stir in the melted margarine until thoroughly combined. Set aside 1 cup of the oat mixture for topping and press the remaining mixture into an ungreased 9×9-inch baking pan. Bake for 20 to 25 minutes, until a knife inserted in the center comes out clean.

Remove the pan from the oven and carefully spread the filling on top of the crust. Sprinkle with the reserved oat mixture. Lightly press the oat mixture into the filling, return to the oven, and bake for 20 to 25 minutes more, until the topping is set. Cool the pan on a wire rack, then cut into bars.

Makes 18 bars

Recipe courtesy of the Oregon Raspberry and Blackberry Commission

Zippy Fruit Dip

One 16-ounce container cottage cheese
1 cup (about 4 ounces) crumbled blue cheese
½ cup chopped walnuts
2 tablespoons honey
Sliced apple, honeydew, and pineapple, to dip

In a small bowl, combine the cottage cheese and blue cheese. Using an electric mixer, beat on high speed until well blended, about 3 minutes. Fold in the walnuts and honey. Cover and refrigerate for 1 to 2 hours to allow the flavors to blend. Serve with apples, honeydew, and pineapple slices to dip.

Makes 6 servings

Recipe courtesy of the Midwest Dairy Association

Creamy Dill Dip

1 cup nonfat sour cream
1 cup nonfat plain yogurt
2 tablespoons dried dill
Cucumber slices, to serve

In a medium bowl, combine the sour cream, yogurt, and dill. If you don't plan to use the dip right away, store it in a covered container until ready to serve. Serve with cucumber slices. To make a creamy salad dressing, add a few tablespoons of water to the dip.

Makes 16 servings

Source: Food Stamp Nutrition Connection

Salmon Spread

One 15½-ounce can salmon
1 tablespoon fresh lemon juice
1 tablespoon bottled horseradish
1 cup plain nonfat yogurt
1 tablespoon dried dill
4 green onions, chopped (or ¼ cup chopped onion or onion
    powder to taste)
Bread, crackers, or rice cakes, to serve
Chopped fresh parsley, to garnish

Drain the salmon and flake with a fork into a medium bowl. Mix in all the other ingredients except the parsley. Serve on bread, crackers, or rice cakes. Sprinkle with the parsley to garnish.

Makes 6 servings

Source: Food Stamp Nutrition Connection

SMART SIDE DISHES

Black and White Bean Salad

1 cup vegetable juice
1 tablespoon vegetable oil
¼ teaspoon garlic powder or 2 cloves garlic, minced
One 15½-ounce can black beans, rinsed and drained
One 15½-ounce can navy beans, rinsed and drained
1 red, yellow, or orange bell pepper, chopped
½ teaspoon onion powder or 1 small onion, chopped
1 cup frozen corn kernels
1 to 2 tablespoons diced green chiles (optional)

In a large bowl or container, combine the vegetable juice, oil, and garlic. Add the beans, bell pepper, onion, corn, and chiles, if using, to the juice mixture and stir to combine. Cover and refrigerate at least 2 hours, or overnight, before serving.

Makes 6 servings

Recipe courtesy of the Northarvest Bean Growers Association

Pesto Sauce

1 medium bunch of basil
4 to 6 tablespoons olive oil
2 cloves garlic, crushed
2 tablespoons pine nuts or walnuts
2 tablespoons grated Parmesan cheese

In a blender or food processor, combine all the ingredients except the cheese and blend until smooth. Stir in the cheese and add more oil if it needs to be thinned out. Serve over pasta.

Makes ¾ cup

Source: Bureau of Markets/Farmers' Markets

Pasta Salad Florentine

6 ounces small tube-shaped pasta
2 tablespoons honey
2½ tablespoons Dijon-style mustard
3 tablespoons red wine vinegar
1½ teaspoons dried oregano
½ teaspoon garlic powder
2 cups (about 2 ounces) torn fresh spinach leaves
2 cups (about 11 ounces) halved cherry tomatoes
1½ cups (about 10 ounces) frozen peas, thawed
½ cup shelled pistachios

Cook the pasta according to the package directions. Drain. To make the dressing, in a medium bowl, whisk together the honey, mustard, vinegar, oregano, and garlic powder. In a large bowl, toss together the pasta, spinach, tomatoes, peas, pistachios, and dressing, until well combined.

Makes 4 servings

Source: Centers for Disease Control

Asian Snow Peas

1 teaspoon sesame oil
½ pound fresh snow peas, trimmed

½ cup diagonally sliced carrot
¼ cup sliced water chestnuts
½ cup low-sodium chicken broth
1 teaspoon low-sodium soy sauce
1 teaspoon cornstarch

Heat the oil in a medium nonstick skillet over medium-high heat until hot. Add the snow peas and carrots and sauté for 2 minutes, or until slightly softened. Add the water chestnuts and chicken broth and bring to a boil. Cover, reduce the heat, and simmer for 5 minutes, or until vegetables are crisp-tender.

In a small bowl, combine the soy sauce and cornstarch, stirring until the cornstarch dissolves. Add to vegetable mixture and cook, stirring constantly, until the sauce thickens. Serve immediately.

Makes 4 servings

Source: Centers for Disease Control

Southwest Cornbread Squares

Nonstick cooking spray
1 box corn muffin mix
1 small onion, thinly sliced
½ cup thinly sliced red bell pepper
½ cup thinly sliced green bell pepper
1 teaspoon dried oregano
1½ cups shredded reduced-fat mild cheddar cheese

Preheat the oven to 400°F. Coat an 8-inch square or round pan with cooking spray.

Prepare the corn muffin mix batter as directed on the

package. Pour the batter into the pan and bake for 15 minutes, or until lightly browned. Remove from the oven but do not remove the cornbread from the pan. Leave the oven on.

While cornbread is baking, heat a medium skillet and coat with cooking spray. Add the onions and bell peppers and sauté until softened, about 5 minutes. Stir in the oregano and set aside.

Sprinkle 1 cup of the cheese over the baked cornbread, then top with the vegetable mixture and remaining ½ cup cheese. Bake for 5 minutes, or until the cheese is melted. Cut the cornbread into 2-inch squares and serve.

Recipe courtesy of the Midwest Dairy Association

BRAIN POWER ENTRÉES

Baked Chicken Nuggets

1 cup cornflakes
½ teaspoon Italian herb seasoning
¼ teaspoon garlic powder
¼ teaspoon onion powder
1 teaspoon paprika
1½ pounds boneless, skinless chicken thighs, cut into bite-size
    pieces

Place the cornflakes in a heavy-duty zip-top bag and crush with a rolling pin. Add the herb seasoning, garlic powder, onion powder, and paprika to the crushed cornflakes. Seal the bag tightly and shake until blended. Add a few chicken pieces at a time to the crumb mixture and shake to coat evenly.

Microwave method: Lightly grease an 8×12-inch baking

dish. Place chicken pieces on baking dish with a little space between them. Cover with wax paper and cook on high until tender, 6 to 8 minutes, rotating the chicken every 2 to 3 minutes.

Oven method: Preheat the oven to 400°F and lightly grease a baking sheet.

Place the chicken pieces on the baking sheet with a little space between them. Place in the oven and bake until golden brown, 12 to 14 minutes.

Makes 4 servings

Source: U.S. Department of Agriculture

Lamb Chops with Cornbread Stuffing

Nonstick cooking spray
Four ¾- to 1-inch-thick lamb shoulder chops (arm or blade)
1⅓ cups water
2 tablespoons unsalted butter or margarine
One 6-ounce package cornbread stuffing mix
One 11-ounce can corn with red and green bell peppers with
    liquid

Spray a large skillet with cooking spray and place over medium-high heat. Cook the chops for 4 to 5 minutes on each side, until browned. Remove the chops from the pan and reduce the heat to low. Add the water, butter, and seasoning packet from the stuffing mix and mix well. Stir in the stuffing mix and corn and liquid. Place the browned chops on top of the stuffing, cover, and cook for 10 to 12 minutes, to desired degree of doneness.

Makes 4 servings

Recipe courtesy of the American Lamb Board

Louisiana Lamb Steaks

1 tablespoon olive oil
1 tablespoon red pepper sauce
Two 1-inch-thick lamb center leg steaks
1 teaspoon coarsely cracked black pepper

Preheat the grill to medium-hot.

In a small bowl, combine the oil and red pepper sauce. Brush the mixture on one side of each steak and sprinkle each with ¼ teaspoon of the pepper, pressing the pepper in with the back of a spoon. Grill the steaks, seasoned side down, 4 inches from the coals for 7 to 10 minutes. Turn and brush with the remaining oil mixture and sprinkle with remaining cracked pepper. Grill for additional 7 to 10 minutes, or to desired degree of doneness: 145°F for medium-rare, 160°F for medium, or 170°F for well done. Cover and let the steaks stand for 10 minutes before cutting and serving. (The internal temperature will rise about 10 degrees.)

Makes 8 servings

Recipe courtesy of the American Lamb Board

Veggie Bean Wrap

2 chopped green or red bell peppers
1 medium onion, sliced
One 15-ounce can black beans, drained and rinsed
2 mangos, peeled, pitted, and chopped
Juice of 1 lime
½ cup chopped fresh cilantro
1 avocado, peeled and diced
Four 10-inch flour tortillas warmed

Heat a nonstick pan over medium heat. Add the bell peppers and onion and sauté for 5 minutes, or until softened. Add the beans and stir well. Reduce the heat to low and simmer about 5 minutes, or until vegetables are tender.

In a medium bowl, combine the mangos, lime juice, cilantro, and avocado. Reserve half of the mixture for topping. Top the warmed tortillas with the bean mixture and remaining mango mixture, dividing evenly. Fold the ends of the tortillas over and roll up to make wraps. Top with the remaining mango mixture.

Makes 4 servings

Source: Food Stamp Nutrition Connection

ENERGIZING DESSERTS

Creamy Rice Pudding

2¾ cups lowfat milk
1 packet Butter Buds Mix, liquefied
½ cup evaporated skim milk
½ cup uncooked long-grain white rice
¼ cup sugar
3 tablespoons cornstarch
1 large egg yolk
¼ cup raisins
3 packets (or 1 teaspoon bulk) Sweet'N Low
1 teaspoon vanilla extract
½ teaspoon ground cinnamon, plus more for sprinkling

In a large saucepan, combine 2 cups of the lowfat milk, the Butter Buds, evaporated skim milk, rice, and sugar. Place over medium heat and bring to a boil. Reduce the heat, cover, and simmer for about 30 minutes, stirring occasionally.

In a small bowl, stir the cornstarch into the remaining ¾ cup lowfat milk and add to the rice mixture. Cook, stirring constantly, until thickened. In a small bowl, beat the egg yolk. Stir in ½ cup of the hot rice mixture, then add back into the saucepan. Cook, stirring constantly, for 1 minute. Add the raisins, Sweet'N Low, vanilla, and cinnamon. Stir until well blended. Pour the pudding into a 12-quart dish. Sprinkle with cinnamon, and cool to room temperature. Serve at room temperature or refrigerate until ready to serve.

Makes 4 servings

Recipe courtesy of the Calorie Control Council

Fresh Blackberry Sundae

2 cups regular or lowfat vanilla ice cream
2 cups fresh blackberries
½ cup whipped topping
4 cherries (optional)

Place ½ cup ice cream in each of 4 sundae dishes. Top each with ½ cup blackberries. Follow with the whipped topping and finish with a cherry, if using.

Makes 4 servings

Recipe courtesy of the North American Bramble Growers Association

Peach-Apple Crisp

One 20-ounce light-syrup packed can sliced peaches,
drained

2 medium tart apples, peeled, cored, and sliced

½ teaspoon vanilla extract

¼ teaspoon ground cinnamon

¾ cup plus 3 tablespoons all-purpose flour

¼ cup packed brown sugar

3 tablespoons margarine, cut into pieces and chilled

Preheat the oven to 350°F. Lightly grease a 9×2-inch casserole dish.

In a large bowl, combine the peaches, apples, vanilla, and cinnamon. Toss well and spread evenly over the casserole dish. In a small bowl, combine the flour and brown sugar. Cut in the margarine with two knives until the mixture resembles coarse meal. Sprinkle the flour mixture evenly over the fruit. Place in the oven and bake until lightly browned and bubbly, about 20 minutes.

Makes 4 servings

Source: U.S. Department of Agriculture

Honey Milk Balls

¼ cup honey

¼ cup creamy peanut butter, any type

½ cup nonfat dry milk

½ cup crushed corn flakes cereal

In a medium bowl, mix together the honey and peanut butter. Gradually add the dry milk and mix well. Chill for easier handling. With greased hands, form the mixture into small balls.

Place the crushed cereal flakes on a large plate and roll the balls into the cereal. Cover and refrigerate until firm. Refrigerate leftovers within 2 hours.

Makes 8 to 10 small balls. Double or triple recipe if you need to serve more.

Source: Food Stamp Nutrition Connection

Sugarless Oatmeal Cookies

Nonstick cooking spray
⅓ cup margarine
3 ripe bananas, cut into pieces
2 cups quick-cooking rolled oats
¼ cup skim milk
½ cup raisins
1 teaspoon vanilla extract

Preheat the oven to 350°F. Coat 2 cookie sheets with cooking spray.

Place the margarine in a small saucepan over low heat and melt it. In a large bowl, combine the remaining ingredients, mixing well. Let stand for about 5 minutes, or until the oats are softened.

Drop tablespoons of the dough onto the cookie sheets. Place in the oven and bake for 15 to 20 minutes, until cookies are very lightly browned. Let the cookies cool on the cookie sheet for about 1 minute, then transfer to wire racks or a dish towel to cool completely.

Makes about 30 cookies

Source: Food Stamp Nutrition Connection

Fat-Free Apple Crumb Dessert

Nonstick cooking spray
4 medium baking apples, peeled, cored, and thinly sliced
½ cup quick-cooking rolled oats
¼ cup light or dark brown sugar
2 teaspoons ground cinnamon
⅓ cup apple juice

Position an oven rack in the center of the oven and preheat the oven to 350°F. Spray the bottom and sides of a 9×13-inch baking dish with cooking spray. Spread the apple slices evenly over the bottom of the baking dish. In a small bowl, use a fork to combine the oats, brown sugar, and cinnamon. Spread the oat mixture evenly over the apples. Evenly pour the apple juice over the oat mixture. Cover with foil, place in the oven, and bake for 20 to 30 minutes, until the apples are just starting to soften. Uncover and bake for another 15 to 20 minutes, until the apples are soft. Cool before serving.

Makes 4 servings

Source: Food Stamp Nutrition Connection

NINE

❋

Fishing for Pain Relief

If you've ever been in pain, you know that it has a way of taking over your life, physically and psychologically. The suffering starts to have a life of its own. The emotional trauma can have an impact on careers, relationships, and dreams. More than 60 million Americans suffer from some kind of chronic pain—pain that persists for six months or more—or from pain stemming from diseases such as arthritis. Pain can take hold, waking up with you in the morning, keeping you awake at night, and lying in wait like a stalker in your body.

Successful treatment depends on a multidisciplinary approach that includes medication, psychological counseling, exercise, and nutrition—an approach usually available through a pain management clinic. The idea behind this type of approach is to tackle pain from every angle so that you can reclaim power over your body. Pain management clinics, developed over the past two decades, teach chronic pain patients how to cope with their pain.

When I (Frank) administered five pain clinics, it was remarkable to note how much diet affected the levels of pain reported by our patients. We conducted an experiment using foods that third world countries were using to manage pain, such as bananas and strawberries. We offered patients one of these foods or sugary ones in their meals. The findings were encouraging. Bananas in particular helped alleviate muscle pain such as spasms. The reason bananas were so beneficial is that they're highly concentrated in natural serotonin, a feel-good chemical also made by the body. Those who chose the sugary foods experienced no relief from their pain.

Nutrition is clearly one tool for pain relief that can help you take back charge of your life. If you're ready to start living with more control over your pain than ever before, here are some specific foods you'll want to add to your diet.

Fish for Pain Relief

Fish is at the top of the nutritional list—again. One of the most promising benefits of fish is found in the treatment of rheumatoid arthritis, a joint disease in which the body's own immune system attacks its tissues. More than 2 million people have this form of arthritis. Most are women.

The chief symptoms of rheumatoid arthritis are pain, swelling, and stiffness—all thought to be triggered by pro-inflammatory chemicals in the body. In a rather dramatic nutritional rescue, omega-3 fatty acids in fish interfere with this inflammatory process and confer an anti-inflammatory effect, which results in less pain and stiffness. In general, eating fish (and taking fish oil supplements) provides moderate pain relief and makes patients less reliant on anti-inflammatory drugs and pain medication.

Here's more good news for your joints: Omega-3 fatty acids may protect you against a more prevalent form of arthritis called osteoarthritis (a joint disease in which cartilage gradually deteriorates). The proof comes from Eskimos, who have the lowest rates of osteoarthritis in the world. They eat a diet rich in fish oils, namely omega-3 fatty acids, which appear to have a protective effect on joints. But in Eskimos who become westernized, the rate of osteoarthritis triples.

To harness the healing power of fish and its beneficial fats, eat two to three four-ounce fish servings a week. Just eating a four-ounce portion of salmon twice a week, for example, serves up about 5 grams of omega-3 fatty acids, the amount recommended by most health care practitioners.

Drizzle Olive Oil, Fizzle Pain

Rich in beneficial monounsaturated fats, olive oil has been used for centuries to maintain the suppleness of the skin, give sheen to hair, and aid in digestion. Ancient Egyptians used olive oil for preserving mummies, and the Bible mentions the oil frequently as a medicine for healing wounds and anointing the sick.

Among unsaturated fats, olive oil stands alone as being resistant to oxidation (toxic changes), a possible factor in heart disease. Because of this attribute, olive oil has been described as the safest fat to eat because it doesn't give off health-damaging free radicals. More recently, olive oil has been shown to conserve heart-protective HDL cholesterol. Further, olive oil seems to guard against certain forms of cancer, specifically cancer of the colon, breast, endometrium, and prostate, as seen in studies of Mediterranean people, who have a lower incidence of these cancers.

Besides the fact that olive oil is a potent source of healthy monounsaturated fats that can help reduce your risk of cardiovascular disease and certain cancers, add yet another benefit to this list: Researchers have found that olive oil acts as a natural pain reliever.

According to a growing body of research, the secret to olive oil's pain-relieving power is a previously unknown ingredient in freshly pressed extra-virgin olive oils, oleocanthal, which acts as an anti-inflammatory, similar to nonsteroidal anti-inflammatory drugs (NSAIDs) such as ibuprofen. In their studies, oleocanthal inhibited the activity of COX-1 and COX-2 (a class of enzymes that make prostaglandins that cause inflammation, pain, and fever) in a manner similar to anti-inflammatory drugs.

Olive oil clearly does your body good. So if you're interested in preventing disease and relieving pain, include olive oil as one of the main healthy fats in your diet.

Fight Pain with Antioxidant-Rich Foods

Fruits and vegetables are loaded with antioxidants, which neutralize free radicals, substances that damage cells. While our bodies constantly produce free radicals, healthy tissues inactivate these damaging substances and keep their levels in check. It's when free-radical production somehow overwhelms the body's natural defenses that problems occur. Studies suggest that antioxidants may fight chronic pain by helping the body to break down free radicals. The study of the pain-killing effects of antioxidants is an emerging area of research. We know already that one antioxidant in particular, vitamin C, works as an anti-inflammatory. Furthermore, it has been found to delay the muscle onset soreness (DOMS) felt in the twenty-four- to forty-eight-hour period following exercise.

An easy way to make sure that you get enough antioxidants is to eat one or more servings a day from each of the following categories of fruits and vegetables: citrus fruits; noncitrus fruits, including berries; green and dark-green leafy vegetables; yellow, orange, or red vegetables such as bell peppers, carrots, and squash; and cruciferous vegetables such as broccoli, Brussels sprouts, and cabbage. Cruciferous vegetables are so named because their re-productive structures contain components that are arranged like a cross; hence the name "cruciferous," which comes from a derivative meaning "to place on a cross," or "crucify."

Enjoy Tropical Fruits

Pineapples contain bromelain, an enzyme thought to block sub-stances responsible for inflammation, swelling, and pain—similar to aspirin. Bromelain has the potential to help reduce joint swell-ing associated with osteoarthritis and rheumatoid arthritis, with many laboratory findings supporting this notion. Additionally, bromelain reduces swelling, bruising, pain, and healing time fol-lowing trauma and surgical procedures. Pineapple also contains beneficial vitamins and minerals, so eating it more frequently to reduce symptoms is certainly worth a try.

Another luscious tropical fruit is papaya. It contains the enzyme papain, also thought to be a strong anti-inflammatory agent. Papaya also contains other enzymes that help break down food in the stomach, which lets you absorb more nutrients. It's also a prebiotic, too, which means it promotes the growth of good bacteria in the gut.

Another pain-relieving fruit is the versatile banana; it works by alleviating anxiety. Feeling anxious can intensify your pain, so anything you can do to calm yourself down naturally—such as reaching for a banana—can help ease your pain.

This chapter includes recipes with foods that soothe pain and restore a feeling of balance. Food truly is medicine—and that includes pain medicine.

SMART TIPS ● PAIN CONTROL

- **BREATHE TO RELIEVE.** Employ deep breathing techniques to help reduce your pain.

- **EASE INTO EXERCISE.** Engage in slow, rhythmic exercises to help relax the tissues around your pain. Yoga is excellent for pain and stress relief.

- **USE MENTAL IMAGERY.** Visualize the space around your pain and imagine that you are putting your pain into a ball or a trap while you allow the rest of your body to relax and unwind.

- **CHANGE YOUR THOUGHT PROCESSES.** Do not play into the victim game of feeling captive to your pain or believing that your pain is a punishment for something you did in the past.

- **ACT TO DISTRACT.** Find ways of distracting yourself from the pain, such as taking short walks, listening to music, or listening to an inspirational message.

continued

- **WATER YOUR BODY AND BRAIN.** Many of the aches and pains we have may be a result of dehydration. For example, a lack of fluid constricts and dilates the blood vessels in the brain, creating a headache.

- **STOP SMOKING.** Smoking makes pain worse. It also interferes with absorption and blood level of various medications, including pain-killers. If you smoke, try to quit or ask your physician for guidance on how to quit.

STARTERS AND OTHER DELIGHTS

Tropical Colada Smoothie

½ cup silken tofu
½ cup chopped fresh mango
½ teaspoon coconut extract
½ cup crushed pineapple (canned in its own juice)
½ cup skim milk
1 tablespoon honey

Place all the ingredients in a blender and blend until smooth. Pour into a glass and serve immediately.

Makes 1 serving

Recipe courtesy of Maggie Greenwood-Robinson

Vanilla Fruit Smoothie

1 cup orange-mango juice
1 packet French Vanilla Carnation Instant Breakfast

¾ cup chopped fresh papaya
3 or 4 ice cubes, crushed

Place all the ingredients in a blender and blend until smooth. Pour into a glass and serve immediately.

Makes 1 serving

Recipe courtesy of Maggie Greenwood-Robinson

Carrot Curls

2 medium carrots
¼ cup blue cheese, softened
½ cup finely chopped celery
¼ cup finely chopped toasted pecans

Halve carrots lengthwise and, using a vegetable peeler along the flat side of each half, cut about 18 long, wide strips. Beginning with the wider end, wind each ribbon around your thumb, securing the ends with wooden picks. Chill the carrot curls in a bowl of ice water for 1 hour.

In a small bowl, cream together the blue cheese, celery, and pecans and drop level teaspoons onto a plate. Cover the filling with plastic and refrigerate for 45 minutes to chill. Drain the carrot curls. Working with 1 carrot curl at a time, remove the wooden pick and pat dry. Beginning with the wider end, wrap each carrot curl around a teaspoon of the filling and resecure the ends with wooden picks.

Makes 18 curls

Recipe courtesy of the Georgia Fruit and Vegetable Growers Association

Hooked on Salmon Sticks

One 14¾-ounce can pink salmon, drained (see Note)
½ cup crushed saltine crackers
1 large egg
Nonstick cooking spray
1 tablespoon olive oil

In a large bowl, combine the salmon, cracker crumbs, and egg. Divide the mixture into 8 pieces and shape into sticks about 4 inches long.

Lightly coat a skillet with cooking spray. Add the oil and heat over medium heat. Add the fish sticks and cook for about 3 minutes, or until golden brown. Flip over and cook for about 3 minutes, or until golden brown.

Makes 8 servings

Note: Canned pink salmon contains soft bones that are a great source of calcium. Take out any large, hard bones, and then mash the small bones with a fork. Once the fish is cooked no one will know the bones are there.

Source: Food Stamp Nutrition Connection

South of the Border Dip

1 cup nonfat sour cream
1 cup nonfat plain yogurt
1 cup prepared salsa
Tortilla chips, crackers, or vegetable sticks, to serve

In a medium bowl, mix together the sour cream, yogurt, and salsa. Serve immediately or cover and store in the refrigerator until ready to serve. Serve with tortilla chips, crackers, or vegetable sticks.

Makes 3 cups of dip

Source: Food Stamp Nutrition Connection

SMART SIDE DISHES

Grapes and Grains

2 tablespoons olive oil

2 tablespoons fresh lemon juice

1 tablespoon orange juice

2 cups cooked barley

1½ cups halved seedless or seeded grapes, any variety

½ cup sliced celery

¼ cup sliced green onions

⅛ teaspoon salt

⅛ teaspoon black pepper

In a large bowl, whisk together the oil, lemon juice, and orange juice. Add the barley, grapes, celery, and green onions, tossing to coat. Season with the salt and pepper. Serve immediately or cover and refrigerate until ready to serve.

Makes 4 servings

Recipe courtesy of the Chilean Fresh Fruit Association

Fruited Squash

3 medium butternut squash, halved and seeds removed

¼ cup water

1 Granny Smith apple, peeled, cored, and cubed
1 cup raisins
1 cup cranraisins
⅔ cup coarsely chopped pecans
¾ cup apple juice
1¼ teaspoons pumpkin pie spice
¼ teaspoon salt
1 tablespoon unsalted butter
1 tablespoon sugar

Preheat the oven to 350°F. Place the squash in an ovenproof dish with the skin side up, add the water, and bake for 45 minutes, or until fork tender. Remove from the oven and set aside. Leave the oven on.

Meanwhile, in a medium saucepan, combine the apple, raisins, cranraisins, pecans, apple juice, and pumpkin pie spice. Place over medium heat, bring to a simmer, and simmer for 10 minutes. Remove from heat and add the salt, butter, and sugar, mixing well to melt the butter. Turn the squash over and stuff with the apple mixture. Return to the oven and bake for additional 10 to 20 minutes, until heated through. Remove from the oven, cut each piece in half, and serve immediately.

Makes 12 servings

Recipe courtesy of the Georgia Fruit and Vegetable Growers Association

Shredded Coleslaw

DRESSING
½ cup light sour cream
½ cup reduced-fat mayonnaise

2 teaspoons celery seeds
1 tablespoon prepared horseradish
¼ teaspoon salt
¼ teaspoon coarsely ground black pepper

SALAD

3 medium carrots, shredded (about 2 cups)
1 medium zucchini, shredded (about 2 cups)
1 small head cabbage, shredded (about 2 cups)
1 medium Vidalia onion, chopped (about 1 cup)

In a small bowl, whisk together the dressing ingredients. Cover and refrigerate for up to 30 minutes.

In a large bowl, stir together the salad ingredients. Cover and refrigerate at least 30 minutes. Drain the salad, pressing out excess moisture. Pour the dressing over the salad and toss to coat well. Serve immediately.

Makes 10 servings

Recipe courtesy of the Georgia Fruit and Vegetable Growers Association

Chutney-Pineapple Slaw

3 tablespoons prepared chutney, any type
½ teaspoon grated orange zest
2 tablespoons fresh orange juice
12½ cups shredded cabbage
½ cup shredded carrot
1 cup coarsely chopped fresh pineapple or 8 ounces pineapple
    tidbits, drained
¼ cup raisins

In a large bowl, combine the chutney, orange zest, and orange juice. Mix well. Add the shredded cabbage, carrot, pineapple, and raisins; toss to mix. Serve immediately or cover and refrigerate until ready to serve.

Makes 10 to 12 large servings

Source: Centers for Disease Control

Roasted Potatoes and Red Onions

4 pounds small red potatoes, peeled and halved
2 large red onions, chopped
2 tablespoons olive oil
1 tablespoon dried parsley, crushed
1 tablespoon dried rosemary, crushed

Preheat the oven to 400°F.

In a large bowl, combine the potatoes and onions. Toss with the oil and seasonings to coat, and spread out over a deep-sided roasting pan. Roast for about 40 minutes, until lightly browned, turning a few times. Serve immediately.

Makes 4 servings

Recipe courtesy of the Pioneer Valley Growers Association

Root Soup

4 small turnips
2 parsnips
2 carrots
2 medium onions

½ cup uncooked barley

6 cups water

2 bouillon cubes, chicken or vegetable

1 tablespoon dried basil

2 dashes of Tabasco sauce

⅛ teaspoon curry powder (optional)

Black pepper

Grate the turnips, parsnips, carrots, and onions by hand or in a food processor. Combine the grated vegetables in a large saucepan. Add the barley, water, bouillon cubes, and basil and bring to a boil. Reduce the heat, cover, and simmer for 1 hour, until vegetables are soft, checking the soup often and adding water as needed. Stir in the Tabasco sauce, curry powder, if using, and pepper.

Makes 4 servings

BRAIN POWER ENTRÉES

Salmon with Fresh Vegetables

Four 6-ounce salmon fillets

MARINADE

⅓ cup olive oil

1 tablespoon balsamic vinegar

3 tablespoons seasoned rice vinegar

1 tablespoon Dijon-style mustard

2 cloves garlic, crushed

½ teaspoon salt

¼ teaspoon coarsely ground black pepper
¼ teaspoon crushed red chile flakes

VEGETABLES

3 cups broccoli florets
1 cup diced plum tomatoes
⅓ cup diced red onion
2 tablespoons capers
2 tablespoons chopped fresh basil leaves
2 tablespoons chopped fresh dill

Rinse the salmon fillets, pat dry, and set aside. To make the marinade, in a small bowl, whisk together all the marinade ingredients. Remove ¼ cup of the marinade to baste the salmon while grilling or broiling.

Steam the broccoli for about 5 minutes, or until crisp-tender. Drain and rinse with cold water. Place in a large bowl and add the tomatoes, onion, capers, basil, and dill. Pour the marinade over the vegetables. Grill or broil the salmon, basting with the reserved marinade, and serve the fish over the vegetables.

Makes 4 servings

Recipe courtesy of the California Salmon Council

Greek-Style Fish with Eggplant

1 medium eggplant
2 teaspoons olive oil

1 cup prepared tomato sauce
¼ cup dry white wine
Juice of 1 lemon
1 tablespoon balsamic vinegar
2 cloves garlic, minced
1 teaspoon dry mustard
1 teaspoon dried oregano
2 tablespoons chopped fresh mint or 1 teaspoon dried mint
1 bay leaf
1 pound fish fillets or 4 small whole trout, cleaned

Preheat the broiler.

Cut the eggplant into ¼-inch-thick slices. Lay the slices in a single layer on the broiling rack. Broil 3 to 4 inches from heat, until the eggplant is browned. Turn and brown on the other side. The eggplant will not be fully cooked.

Set the oven to 375°F. In a medium saucepan, combine all the remaining ingredients except the fish. Place over medium heat, bring to a boil, then reduce the heat to very low, and simmer, uncovered, for 15 minutes, or until the sauce is thick.

Arrange the grilled eggplant slices in an overlapping pattern in an ovenproof dish or shallow casserole. Lay the fish on top of the eggplant. Spread the sauce over the fish. Bake for 10 minutes, or until the fish is cooked through. Serve immediately.

Makes 4 servings

Recipe courtesy of the Chilean Fresh Fruit Association

Sea Bass with Nectarine Salsa

Four 7-ounce Chilean sea bass fillets
Salt
1 cup unsweetened coconut milk
5 tablespoons fresh lime juice
1 tablespoon curry powder
2 cups finely chopped ripe nectarines
3 tablespoons chopped pasilla or poblano chile
1 tablespoon chopped fresh cilantro
1 tablespoon chopped fresh mint
Lime wedges and fresh mint sprigs, to garnish
Cooked rice, to serve (optional)

Preheat the oven to 350°F. Arrange the sea bass in an oven-proof dish in one layer. Season with salt to taste. In small bowl, combine the coconut milk, 1 tablespoon of the lime juice, and the curry powder and pour over the fish. Cover and bake for 15 to 25 minutes, depending on the thickness of the fish, until cooked through.

To make the salsa, in a medium bowl, combine the nectarines, chile, cilantro, mint, and remaining 4 tablespoons lime juice.

To serve, arrange the sea bass on individual plates, spoon the curry sauce over, and top with the salsa. Garnish with lime wedges and fresh mint sprigs. Serve with rice, if you like.

Makes 4 servings

Recipe courtesy of the Chilean Fresh Fruit Association

Buttery Shrimp and Eggplant Kabobs

1 tablespoon whipped butter, melted
1 tablespoon chopped fresh basil
2 teaspoons olive oil
2 cloves garlic, minced
1 teaspoon fresh lemon juice
Dash of black pepper
7 ounces peeled and deveined large shrimp
½ cup halved eggplant slices
Lettuce, basil sprigs, and lemon wedges, to garnish (optional)

In a medium bowl, combine all the ingredients except the shrimp and eggplant and stir to combine. Add the shrimp and eggplant and turn to coat. Cover and refrigerate at least 1 hour or overnight.

Preheat the barbecue or a gas grill on high. Alternately thread half of the shrimp and eggplant onto each of two 12-inch or four 6-inch metal or presoaked bamboo skewers.

Place the kabobs on the rack and cook for 4 to 6 minutes, turning occasionally and basting with the marinade until shrimp turn pink. Serve, garnished with lettuce, basil, and lemon, if you like.

Makes 4 servings

Recipe courtesy of Andrea Laudate

Quick Catfish Creole

1 pound catfish fillets
One 24-ounce jar mild chunky salsa
Rice, to serve

Preheat the oven to 400°F.

Place the fish in an ungreased baking dish. Pour the salsa over fish. Bake, uncovered, for 25 minutes, or until the fish flakes easily with a fork. Serve over rice.

Makes 4 servings

Recipe courtesy of Maggie Greenwood-Robinson

ENERGIZING DESSERTS

Papaya Cake

½ cup vegetable shortening

1½ cups sugar

2 large eggs

2 cups diced fresh papaya

3 cups all-purpose flour

2 teaspoons baking soda

1 teaspoon salt

1 teaspoon ground cinnamon

½ teaspoon ground nutmeg

¼ teaspoon ground ginger

2 tablespoons water

1 teaspoon fresh lemon juice

1 cup raisins

Preheat the oven to 350°F. Grease and flour a 9×13-inch baking pan.

In the large bowl of an electric mixer, cream together the shortening and sugar. Add the eggs, one at a time, beating well after each addition. Add the papaya and beat well. In a separate bowl, sift the flour with the baking soda, salt, cinnamon, nutmeg, and ginger. Stir into the papaya mixture. Add the water and lemon juice and fold in the raisins.

Pour into the prepared pan, place in the oven, and bake for 40 to 50 minutes, until knife inserted in the center comes out clean.

Makes 16 servings

Recipe courtesy of the Hawaii Papaya Industry Association

Fruit Mix

½ cup unpeeled diced apple
½ cup sliced banana
½ cup cut-up grapefruit sections
2 tablespoons grapefruit juice or pineapple juice
⅓ cup halved grapes
⅓ cup juice-packed pineapple tidbits

In a medium bowl, combine the apple, banana, grapefruit, and grapefruit juice. Add the grapes and pineapple. Cover and refrigerate to chill.

Makes 2 servings

Source: Centers for Disease Control

Hawaiian Ambrosia

One 20-ounce can pineapple chunks, in natural juice
One 11-ounce can mandarin oranges
One 17-ounce can fruit cocktail
½ cup shredded unsweetened coconut flakes
1 cup nonfat plain yogurt or sour cream

1 cup miniature marshmallows
½ cup raisins
¼ cup pecans

Drain the canned fruit well and place in a large bowl. Add the coconut, yogurt, marshmallows, raisins, and pecans. Mix well, cover, and refrigerate for 1 hour before serving.

Makes 8 servings

Source: Centers for Disease Control

Frozen Fruit Pops

8 ounces crushed pineapple, canned in its own juice
1 cup lowfat fruit yogurt
6 ounces frozen orange juice concentrate, thawed

In a medium bowl, mix together all the ingredients. Divide into 4 paper cups and freeze until slushy, about 1 hour. Insert a wooden stick halfway through the center of each fruit pop, then freeze until hard, at least 4 hours. Peel away the paper cups and serve. Alternatively, you can freeze the mixture in ice cube trays to make fruit-flavored ice cubes to serve in fruit juice.

Makes 4 servings

Source: Food Stamp Nutrition Connection

Pineapple-Orange Frozen Yogurt

1 cup nonfat vanilla yogurt
1 cup canned pineapple chunks in their own juice
½ cup orange juice

Place the yogurt and fruit in a large zip-top bag, flatten, and freeze overnight. In a food processor or blender, combine the fruit and yogurt mixture with the orange juice and process until smooth. Serve immediately or place back in the freezer for up to 1 hour to harden, stirring occasionally. Stir just before serving.

Makes 4 servings

Source: Food Stamp Nutrition Connection

TEN

※

Be a Smart, Creative Eater

Whether it's dreaming up a new product or figuring out what to serve for dinner, creative thinking is a part of life, and you don't have to be an artist or a poet or musician to need it. Creativity is behind every business success, every work of architecture, every scrumptious meal at your favorite restaurant, and more.

But can you eat your way to higher intelligence and greater creativity? Quite possibly, and many of the nutrients we've discussed throughout this book—like omega-3 oils—are now being touted as intelligence boosters. Recent research suggests they help the circulation system that pumps oxygen to your head, as well as improve the function of the membranes that surround brain cells. A few years ago, we developed a special nutritional program for business leaders that involved having them fast for three days with only water and fruit to help cleanse the body and brain from toxins so that thoughts would not be hindered. Then we put them on a diet that included grilled fish dishes such as salmon and tuna and high-fiber foods. In measuring their creativity before and after the diet, we found that the special diet of detoxing and eating more fish improved creativity.

In addition to fish, other types of protein are valuable to your brain for needle-sharp thinking throughout the day. Protein helps the brain synthesize neurotransmitters; builds and repairs tissues; keeps your immune system functioning up to par; helps carry nutrients throughout your body; and has a hand in forming hormones. You simply must have a protein-rich diet to stay mentally focused and creative. Case in point: Kira, a client, had dreams of becoming a writer, but her manuscripts had been rejected consistently. Her diet wasn't helping matters; she snacked on processed foods, commercial cupcakes, and other sugar-laced foods. She was overweight by nearly one hundred pounds as a result. Once she switched to a diet that included grilled chicken and fish, eggs, and plenty of vegetables, everything changed. She finally finished, and published, a series of children's books— and lost sixty pounds in the process.

When I (Frank) begin the process of writing a book, I make my own creativity booster. It consists of two raw fresh eggs, a banana, supplements of B_{12}, B_6, and gingko, a scoop of chocolate protein powder, water, and ice. I blend them all together for a few seconds until the ice is mushy and my thought process feels turbocharged. Your diet does change how creatively you think.

Here's more food for thought.

Feed Your Kids Well

Strive to prepare meals for your family that are made from natural, wholesome foods, particularly those free of preservatives, dyes, and colorings. In a fascinating study of 1 million schoolchildren in the New York City school system, there was a 14 percent improvement in IQ scores after additives, preservatives, dyes, artificial flavorings, and colorings were removed from their lunches. So an important factor in improving IQ scores among kids is healthy nutrition.

Fortify Your Diet with Iron-Rich Foods

Iron is a vital mineral for the healthy upkeep of your central nervous system, which includes the brain and spinal cord. When iron is in good supply, you'll think more clearly, be able to retain more information, and learn new tasks easily. With the exception of some fortified foods, liver is the richest source of iron, but if you can't stomach the taste of it, lean beef is your next best bet. Poultry such as chicken and goose contain appreciable amounts, too. Vegetarians can obtain iron through broccoli and green leafy vegetables and dried fruits such as raisins, figs, and apricots. If you eat foods rich in vitamin C (such as oranges, citrus juice, or bell peppers), your body will absorb iron more readily. For example, you can enjoy some orange juice in the morning with a bowl of iron-fortified cereal.

Enjoy Soy

Soy foods such a soybeans, soy flour, and tofu have so much going for them that it's hard to argue that we don't need at least a little soy in our diets. Soy phytoestrogens (natural estrogenlike compounds in soy) may act on the nervous system, affecting mood, cognitive function (including creativity), and behavior. In addition, several studies suggest that soy phytoestrogens protect the brain from damage. Soy provides a complete source of dietary protein, meaning that, unlike most plant proteins, it contains all the essential amino acids. This near-miracle food may also increase glucose uptake in several regions of the brain, and with more glucose, the brain simply functions more clearly and creatively.

Because soy has favorable effects on cholesterol, we know that it is linked to a lower risk of cardiovascular disease, which bodes well for the brain because what is good for the heart is also good for the brain. Soy is so good for cardiovascular health that the FDA suggests that 25 grams of soy protein a day, along with a diet low in saturated fat and cholesterol, may reduce the risk of heart disease. Twenty-five grams is roughly what you'd get in a cup of cooked soybeans or a cup of tofu.

Jump-Start with Java

The cup of coffee or tea you enjoy every morning contains one of the most amazing creativity boosters ever: caffeine. Caffeine not only gets you going in the morning; it boosts your mental powers. Technically, caffeine is a drug—in fact, the most widely used drug in the world.

After drinking a cup of coffee, you'll be able to think more clearly, and your imagination will be stimulated by the caffeine. These positive effects have been confirmed time after time in a number of laboratory tests in which caffeine has been shown to radically improve performance on cognitive tests.

If you want the mental kick that coffee or tea gives, how much should you drink? About one or two cups is all it takes; more than that and you're apt to get too jittery to focus. Caffeine may aggravate certain health problems such as ulcers, heart disease, and high blood pressure, to name just a few.

Here are some delicious recipes to incorporate into your diet that will help give you the creative edge you're looking for.

SMART TIPS ● CREATIVITY BUILDERS

- Learn how to breathe so that your brain gets maximum oxygen—12 to 14 respirations per minute.

- Play games that challenge your mind. Competitive games are often more fun.

- Take a class on a subject you've never studied, or take a creativity workshop.

- Keep a notebook around and write notes to yourself about interesting ideas or events that come to you.

- Study a problem intensely, then sleep on it. Your subconscious goes to work while you're sleeping, and you'll have your creative solution the next morning.

- Try to write down your dreams as soon as you can so you don't forget them.

- Give yourself a specific time each day, uninterrupted, to just allow your creativity to flow.

STARTERS AND OTHER DELIGHTS

Café Mexicano

4 teaspoons chocolate syrup
½ cup heavy cream
¾ teaspoon ground cinnamon
¼ teaspoon ground nutmeg
1 tablespoon sugar
1½ cups strong hot coffee

Put 1 teaspoon of the chocolate syrup into each of 4 coffee cups. In a medium bowl, combine the heavy cream, ¼ teaspoon of the cinnamon, the nutmeg, and sugar and using an electric mixer beat until soft peaks form. Stir the remaining ½ teaspoon cinnamon into the hot coffee. Divide the coffee equally among the 4 cups and stir to blend the coffee with the chocolate syrup. Top with the spiced whipped cream and serve immediately.

Makes 4 servings

Recipe courtesy of the National Coffee Association of U.S.A., Inc.

Ice Cream Parlor Mocha Sodas

½ cup hot water
8 teaspoons finely ground coffee beans
2 cups milk
4 scoops chocolate ice cream
1 quart club soda
Sweetened whipped cream or prepared whipped topping, to serve

Place the hot water in a medium pitcher. Add the coffee and stir until dissolved. Stir in the milk. Place 1 scoop of ice cream in each of 4 ice cream soda glasses. Divide the coffee-milk mixture equally among the glasses and fill the glasses almost to the brim with club soda. Top with whipped cream and serve immediately.

Makes 4 servings

Recipe courtesy of the National Coffee Association of U.S.A., Inc.

Blueberry Pancakes

1½ cups soy flour
2¼ cups all-purpose flour
3 tablespoons plus 1 teaspoon baking powder
¼ cup sugar
1½ teaspoons salt
3 large eggs
3 cups vanilla soymilk
4 tablespoons vegetable oil
2 cups fresh or frozen unthawed blueberries
Nonstick cooking spray

In a large bowl, mix together all the ingredients until well combined. Spray a skillet or griddle with nonstick cooking spray and heat over medium-high heat. Pour the pancake batter on the griddle ½ cup at a time. When bubbles appear on top, flip and cook the other side, until lightly browned and cooked through.

Makes 12 large pancakes

Recipe courtesy of Revival Soy

Soynut Trail Mix

1 cup roasted, salted soynuts
1½ cups candy-coated soynuts
1 cup O-shaped cereal
2 cups frosted mini wheat square cereal
1 cup raisins
1 cup dried cranberries
½ cup dried unsweetened cherries

In a large bowl or container, mix together all the ingredients. Keep tightly closed in the container or a zip-top plastic bag.

Makes 16 servings

Recipe courtesy of Revival Soy

Chipotle Chile Dip

1 teaspoon Chipotle Tabasco sauce
Two 8-ounce containers lowfat plain yogurt
½ cup thick and chunky salsa
2 tablespoons chopped fresh cilantro
¼ cup shredded cheddar cheese
Assorted cut-up vegetables or corn chips, to serve

In a medium bowl, combine all the ingredients except the cheese. Mix until will blended, cover, and refrigerate for 2 hours. Just before serving, add the shredded cheese. Serve with vegetables or corn chips.

Makes 3 cups of dip

Recipe courtesy of Dairy Management Inc.

SMART SIDE DISHES

Broccoli Salad

6 cups chopped broccoli florets

1 cup raisins

1 medium red onion, diced

2 tablespoons sugar

8 bacon slices, cooked and crumbled (optional)

2 tablespoons fresh lemon juice

¾ cup reduced-fat mayonnaise

In a medium bowl, combine all the ingredients and mix well. Cover and refrigerate for 1 to 2 hours before serving.

Makes 4 servings

Source: Food Stamp Nutrition Connection

California Fig and Citrus Salad

DRESSING

⅓ cup orange juice

2 tablespoons balsamic vinegar

2 tablespoons olive oil

1 tablespoon honey

¼ teaspoon salt

⅛ teaspoon red chile flakes

SALAD

2 navel oranges, peeled and sliced crosswise

8 large fresh black or green figs, sliced lengthwise ¼ inch thick

1 small red onion, thinly sliced
Spinach leaves, to serve
⅓ cup chopped, toasted walnuts

To make the dressing, in a blender, combine the orange juice, vinegar, oil, honey, salt, and chile flakes. Blend until thoroughly combined. Place the oranges, figs, and onion in a large bowl and toss to coat with the dressing. Set aside for at least 10 minutes or up to 1 hour.

To serve, line individual salad plates with spinach leaves. Spoon the salad on top, dividing equally. Top the salads with the walnuts.

Makes 4 servings

Recipe courtesy of the California Fresh Fig Growers Association

Spring Watermelon Salad with Citrus Vinaigrette

SALAD

6 cups watercress (leaves and tops of stems)
4 cups cubed seedless watermelon
½ cup chopped green onion
½ cup chopped fresh chervil leaves (optional)
¼ cup chopped flat-leaf parsley
½ teaspoon sesame oil
3 tablespoons sesame seeds

CITRUS VINAIGRETTE

½ cup olive oil
½ cup peanut oil
3 tablespoons minced shallot

2 tablespoons rice vinegar

2 tablespoons cider vinegar

1 tablespoon fresh orange juice

1 tablespoon fresh lemon juice

1 tablespoon fresh lime juice

2 teaspoons coarse-grain Dijon-style mustard

1 teaspoon honey

To make the salad, in a large bowl, toss together the watercress, watermelon, green onion, chervil, if using, and parsley. Set aside. Heat the sesame oil in a small skillet over low heat. Add the sesame seeds and cook, stirring, until they just begin to darken. Remove from the heat, let cool, and toss with the watermelon mixture. Cover with plastic wrap and refrigerate until ready to serve.

To make the vinaigrette, place all the vinaigrette ingredients in a blender or food processor and blend until smooth. Pour ⅓ cup of the vinaigrette over the salad, toss to coat, and serve immediately.

Makes 6 servings

Recipe courtesy of the National Watermelon Promotion Board's
Director of Communications

Baked Beans

6 cups cooked great Northern or navy beans

3 cups cooked soybeans

1 cup chopped onion

1 cup chopped green bell pepper

2 cloves garlic, minced

Two 8-ounce cans tomato sauce

3 tablespoons molasses

3 tablespoons brown sugar

1 tablespoon cider vinegar

1 teaspoon prepared mustard

1 teaspoon ground ginger

¼ teaspoon ground cinnamon

¼ teaspoon ground allspice

¼ teaspoon black pepper

In a 3-quart casserole, combine all the ingredients. Cover the casserole, turn the oven to 325°F (no need to preheat), and bake for 1 hour. Remove the cover, stir the beans, and bake for about 30 minutes longer.

Makes 18 servings

Recipe courtesy of Revival Soy

Mexican Black Soybean and Corn Salad

Two 15-ounce cans black soybeans, drained and rinsed

2 cups frozen corn kernels, thawed

1 large red bell pepper, chopped

½ cup chopped red onion

1 cup chopped green onions

1 jalapeño chile, minced

2 medium tomatoes, chopped

⅔ cup chopped fresh cilantro

1 tablespoon olive oil

Juice of 2 limes (about ¼ cup)

1½ teaspoons minced garlic
1½ teaspoons ground cumin
1 teaspoon salt

In a large bowl, combine the soybeans, corn, bell pepper, red onion, green onion, chile, tomatoes, and cilantro. Make the dressing by whisking together the oil, lime juice, garlic, cumin, and salt in a medium bowl. Pour over the salad and toss lightly to combine. Cover and refrigerate for at least 2 hours before serving.

Makes 10 servings

Recipe courtesy of Revival Soy

Colby Cobb Salad

DRESSING

2 cups nonfat plain yogurt
4 large basil leaves
¼ cup chopped fresh parsley
2 tablespoons chopped fresh chives
1 tablespoon fresh lemon juice
1 teaspoon honey
½ teaspoon salt
⅛ to ⅜ teaspoon black pepper, to taste
2 tablespoons reduced-fat mayonnaise

SALAD

8 cups chopped romaine lettuce (about 1 small head)
½ cup halved cherry or grape tomatoes
¼ cup thinly sliced red onion

1 cup diced cucumber

2 slices cooked turkey breast, cut into strips

2 tablespoons bacon bits

1 hard-cooked egg, chopped

1½ cups shredded Colby or Colby Jack cheese

To make the dressing, place 1 cup of the yogurt, basil, parsley, chives, lemon juice, honey, salt, and pepper in a blender or food processor and pulse until smooth. Pour the yogurt mixture into a medium bowl and stir in the remaining 1 cup yogurt and the mayonnaise until just blended. Refrigerate until ready to serve. The dressing may be prepared up to 2 days ahead and stored in an airtight container in the refrigerator.

To make the salad, place the lettuce at the bottom of a serving bowl and add the tomatoes, onion, cucumber, turkey, bacon bits, egg, and cheese. Just before serving, pour the dressing over the salad and toss lightly.

Makes 6 servings

Recipe courtesy of Dairy Management Inc.

BRAIN POWER ENTRÉES

Barbecued Chicken

5 tablespoons tomato paste

1 teaspoon ketchup

2 teaspoons honey

1 teaspoon molasses

1 teaspoon Worcestershire sauce

4 teaspoons white vinegar
¾ teaspoon cayenne pepper
⅛ teaspoon black pepper
¼ teaspoon onion powder
2 cloves garlic, minced
⅛ teaspoon grated ginger
1½ pounds (breasts and drumsticks) skinless chicken

In a large saucepan, whisk together all the ingredients except the chicken. Place over medium heat, bring to a simmer, and simmer for 15 minutes.

Wash the chicken and pat dry with paper towels. Place on a large platter and brush with half of the marinade. Cover with plastic wrap and marinate in the refrigerator for 1 hour.

Preheat the broiler. Remove the chicken from the refrigerator, place it on a baking sheet lined with foil, and broil for 10 minutes on each side to seal in the juices. Turn down the oven to 350°F and add the remaining sauce to the chicken and turn to coat. Cover with foil and bake for 30 minutes, or until chicken is cooked throughout.

Makes 4 servings

A Healthier You, www.health.gov

Chicken Salad

3 tablespoons reduced-fat mayonnaise
1 tablespoon fresh lemon juice
¼ cup chopped celery
½ teaspoon onion powder

⅛ *teaspoon salt*

3¼ *cups cubed cooked, skinless chicken*

In a large bowl, combine the mayonnaise, lemon juice, celery, onion powder, and salt. Add the chicken and mix well.

Makes 5 servings

Source: Department of Health and Human Services

Roast Goose with Baked Apple

One 8-pound goose, cleaned, giblets reserved

2 tablespoons vegetable oil

2 cups breadcrumbs

1 medium onion, chopped

¼ *teaspoon dried sage*

1 teaspoon salt

Pinch of black pepper

8 apples

¼ *cup brown sugar*

3 medium sweet potatoes, cooked and mashed

Sauté the giblets in 2 tablespoons vegetable oil until tender, cool, chop, and set aside.

Make the stuffing by combining the breadcrumbs, onion, sage, salt, pepper, and giblets. Stuff the goose with the stuffing and sew together the neck and back.

Roast for about 3 hours, or until goose is done throughout. Core the apples, sprinkle with the brown sugar, and stuff with the mashed sweet potatoes. Place on a baking sheet and bake until tender. Remove from the oven, carve the goose, and serve.

Makes 8 to 10 servings

Recipe courtesy of the Nevada Waterfowl Association

Easy Lasagna

8 ounces button mushrooms, chopped
1½ cups chopped zucchini
16 ounces firm tofu, drained
1 tablespoon fresh lemon juice
1 tablespoon dried parsley flakes
1 teaspoon Italian herb seasoning
¼ teaspoon black pepper
4 cups fat-free prepared marinara sauce
¾ cup water
8 ounces uncooked lasagna noodles
4 ounces mozzarella-style soy cheese, grated
¼ cup Parmesan-style soy cheese

Preheat the oven to 350°F.

Place the mushrooms and zucchini in a large nonstick skillet. Place over medium heat and cook until tender, about 5 minutes, adding a little water if needed. Remove from the heat and set aside. In a medium bowl, mash the tofu with a potato masher. Add the lemon juice, parsley flakes, herb seasoning, and pepper and mix well. Combine the marinara sauce and water. (The extra water will be absorbed by the uncooked noodles.)

To assemble the lasagna, spread about a third of the sauce over the bottom of a 9×13-baking dish. Top with half of the uncooked noodles, half the tofu mixture, half the soy cheese, and all of the mushrooms and zucchini. Place another third of the sauce on top, followed by the remaining noodles, the remaining tofu, and the last third of the sauce. Top with the remaining mozzarella and Parmesan cheeses. Cover with foil and bake at 350°F for 1 hour, or until bubbly and lightly browned. Remove from the oven and let sit for 10 to 15 minutes before serving. Cut the lasagna into 18 pieces and serve.

Makes 9 servings

Recipe courtesy of Revival Soy

Beef Pot Roast

1 beef bouillon cube
2 cups plus 2 tablespoons hot water
1 tablespoon orange juice
¼ teaspoon ground allspice
⅛ teaspoon black pepper
½ cup chopped onion
2½ pounds boneless beef chuck roast

In a small bowl, dissolve the bouillon cube in the 2 cups hot water. In a medium bowl, stir together the broth, orange juice, allspice, and pepper. Heat the 2 tablespoons water in a deep saucepan over medium heat. Add the onion, and cook it until softened, about 5 minutes. Raise the heat, add the roast to the skillet, and brown on all sides. Pour the broth over the meat, bring to a simmer, then reduce the heat and simmer for 2 hours.

Makes 8 servings

Source: U.S. Department of Agriculture

Meaty Stuffed Potatoes

4 large Russet potatoes
¾ cup skim milk
1 tablespoon all-purpose flour
¼ teaspoon black pepper
Nonstick cooking spray
1 cup diced, cooked turkey, chicken, beef, or pork
1 cup coarsely chopped broccoli
½ cup chopped onion
½ cup thinly sliced carrot
¾ cup hot water
½ cup shredded lowfat cheddar cheese

Cut the potatoes in half and place in a medium saucepan. Add just enough water to cover. Place over medium-high heat, bring to a boil, and cook until fork-tender, 15 to 20 minutes. Remove from the heat and drain. Set aside. (Alternatively, you can pierce the whole potatoes in several places with a knife or fork and cook in the microwave without water until fork-tender, then cut each in half.)

Meanwhile, in a jar with a tight-fitting lid, combine the milk, flour, and pepper and shake well to dissolve the flour. Coat a large skillet with cooking spray. Add the meat, broccoli, onion, carrots, and water. Place over medium-high heat, bring to a simmer, then reduce the heat and cook until the vegetables are fork-tender, about 5 minutes. Reduce the heat to low, stir the flour mixture into the meat mixture until well blended, then stir in the cheese. Cook, stirring frequently, for about 5 minutes longer, or until the sauce thickens.

To serve, place 2 potato halves on each plate and mash the middle a little with a fork. Spoon about ⅓ cup of the meat mixture over each potato half and serve.

Makes 4 servings

Source: Food Stamp Nutrition Connection

ENERGIZING DESSERTS

Almond Coffee Cream

2 teaspoons finely ground coffee beans
¼ cup skim milk
2 large egg whites
½ teaspoon salt
Low-calorie sugar substitute equal to ¼ cup sugar
⅛ teaspoon almond extract
¼ cup finely chopped almonds, plus more to garnish (optional)
½ cup nondairy whipped topping

In a small bowl, dissolve the coffee in the milk and set aside.

In a medium bowl, using an electric mixer, combine the egg whites and salt and beat until foamy. Gradually add the sugar substitute and continue to beat until the mixture forms stiff, shiny peaks. Blend in the coffee-milk mixture, almond extract, and chopped almonds. Fold in the whipped topping. Spoon into 6 parfait glasses, and freeze until firm. Garnish with additional chopped almonds, if using.

Makes 6 servings

Recipe courtesy of the National Coffee Association of U.S.A., Inc.

Tapioca Pudding with Mango Sauce

PUDDING
⅓ cup sugar
3 tablespoons minute tapioca
2¾ cups lowfat milk
1 large egg white
1 teaspoon vanilla extract

MANGO SAUCE
½ cup lowfat vanilla yogurt
½ cup mango sorbet

Prepare the tapioca according to the package directions. Cool. In a medium bowl, combine the yogurt and mango sorbet. Mix well.

Layer the pudding in 4 tall wine glasses alternating with the mango sauce. Serve cold.

Makes 4 servings

Recipe courtesy of Dairy Management Inc.

Key Lime Cheesecake

One 11-ounce box no-bake cheesecake mix
One 12-ounce package firm silken tofu
5 tablespoons fresh or bottled lime juice
2 tablespoons fresh lime zest

Make the crust according to package directions for the cheesecake mix. Press firmly against the sides of pie plate first using your fingers or a large spoon to shape the edges. Press the remaining crumbs firmly on the bottom using your hands or a measuring cup.

To make the filling, in a food processor or blender combine the tofu, lime juice, and lime zest and process until smooth and creamy. The filling will be thick. Spoon the filling into the crust, cover with plastic, and refrigerate for at least 1 hour before slicing.

Makes 8 servings

Recipe courtesy of Revival Soy

Praline Pumpkin Pie

FILLING

One 12-ounce package firm silken tofu
1 cup sour cream
One 15-ounce can pure pumpkin
1 cup firmly packed light brown sugar
1 large egg
1 tablespoon all-purpose flour
1 tablespoon pumpkin pie spice
½ teaspoon salt
One 9-inch unbaked pastry shell

PRALINE TOPPING

1 cup chopped pecans
¼ cup firmly packed light brown sugar
3 tablespoons margarine, melted

Preheat the oven to 425°F.

In a food processor or blender, combine the tofu, sour cream, pumpkin, brown sugar, egg, flour, pumpkin pie spice, and salt and process until smooth. Pour into the pastry shell and bake for 15 minutes. Reduce the oven temperature to 350°F and bake for an additional 40 minutes.

While the pie is baking, make the praline topping: In a small bowl, combine the pecans, light brown sugar, and margarine. Sprinkle the praline topping around the edges of pie and bake for 10 minutes longer. Cool, then slice.

Makes 8 servings

Recipe courtesy of Revival Soy

ELEVEN

❄️

Aphrodisiac Foods

Even before French queens tried to turn themselves on for their kings by living on truffles, vanilla, and celery, food and romance were, well, intimate. Nearly every food, from artichoke to avocado, has been considered an aphrodisiac. The ancient Romans were said to prefer such exotic aphrodisiacs as hippo snouts and hyena eyeballs, and traditional Chinese medicine espoused the use of rare delicacies such as rhino horn.

Named after Aphrodite, the Greek goddess of sexual love and beauty, an aphrodisiac is a food, drink, drug, scent, or device that supposedly has powers to increase sexual desire, or libido. Foods that are exotic or suggestive of certain body parts are especially desirable as aphrodisiacs. The avocado tree, for example, was called a "testicle tree" by the Aztecs because its fruit hangs in pairs on the tree, resembling the male testicles. Its aphrodisiac value is based on this resemblance. The phallus-shaped carrot has been associated with sexual stimulation since ancient times and was used by early Middle Eastern royalty to aid in seduction. The fig is another fruit that has claims to aphrodisiac qualities based on its appearance. An open fig is thought to look similar to the female sex organs.

If you consider the food-brain connection, there may be a lot to this aphrodisiac business. After all, the brain is your biggest sex organ, and if you are preoccupied mentally with other issues, it can affect your ability to enjoy sex and achieve an orgasm. In reality, your mind is doing most of the work. Bottom line: Like so many aspects of brain health, your sex drive is affected by what you put into your body.

The use of food as an aphrodisiac may be more truth than myth. Take the myth that oysters are an aphrodisiac, for example. Oysters were first called aphrodisiacs by the ancient Romans, who wrote about the immoral behavior of women who ate them. For one thing, oysters have high zinc levels, which are supposed to increase sperm count. For another, they're high in omega-3 fatty acids, which make your nervous system function better. The banana is another example. Considered an aphrodisiac because of its phallic shape, bananas are rich in potassium and B vitamins, which are said to be necessary for sex-hormone production.

There's more: A healthy diet promotes weight loss and thus holds libido-boosting potential. Obesity is a known risk factor for erectile dysfunction and low testosterone, so peeling off pounds can help pump out more testosterone, and thus enhance sexual function. Slimming down simply makes anyone, man or woman, feel better about themselves and sexually more desirable.

Myth or truth? Maybe foods really do deliver. If so, here are some foods that may kick-start your love life.

Grab Some Granola

Leonardo da Vinci, through his dissection of the penises of cadavers, was the first scientist to realize that during an erection the male sex organ fills with blood. Today it's well known scientifically that better circulation to the extremities results in greater erectile response and an increased sexual response in women. One nutrient that has been found to help is the amino acid arginine. Though you can get it in supplements, arginine is also plentiful in granola, oats, peanuts, cashews, walnuts, dairy, green vegetables, root vegetables, garlic, ginseng, soybeans, and chickpeas.

Good Fats Are Good for Sex

Another way to increase blood flow is through your choice of dietary fats. From an erection standpoint, anything that's good for your heart is good for your penis. Too much saturated fat can, over time, clog arteries and, in doing so, prevent an adequate flow of blood from reaching the genital region. This not only interferes with the ability to perform, but also with sexual pleasure.

Too little fat, on the other hand, is also bad. Your body requires fat to produce your hormones, including the sex hormones testosterone and estrogen. Both are needed for a healthy sex drive. To make sure you get enough fat, choose healthy fats in moderate amounts (no more than a couple of teaspoons a day). Some examples include olive oil, canola oil, walnut oil, nuts, seeds, and fats found in fish.

For a Good Time, Try Soy

Soy, cultivated for more than three thousand years, is both a drug and a food. It contains isoflavones, which help the vaginal area remain lubricated. However, it's important to note that women who have a history of breast cancer should not eat large amounts of soy, because its estrogenlike characteristics may actually increase the risk of reoccurrence. As for men, studies have shown that soy is also beneficial to the prostate, a crucial male sex organ. Among the most popular soy foods are soymilk, soy cheese, tofu, soy meat (made from textured soy in granule form). Most of these products are soy flour derivatives, while tofu is obtained by curdling soymilk.

Pile on Some Papaya

Like soy, papaya is estrogenic, meaning it has compounds that act as the female hormone estrogen. It has been used as a folk remedy in promoting menstruation and milk production, facilitating childbirth, and increasing the female libido.

SMART TIPS ● SPICE UP YOUR LOVE LIFE

Your menu to jazz up your lovemaking should also include spices. Down through the ages, many spices and herbs have been known to help lovers get in the mood. Here's a look.

BASIL (SWEET BASIL). For centuries basil has been believed to rev up sex drive and boost fertility, as well as produce a general sense of well-being. The scent of basil was said to drive men wild—so much so that women would dust their breasts with dried and powdered basil. Basil also may help promote circulation.

CARDAMOM. Cultures throughout the world have deemed cardamom a powerful treatment for impotence. It is high in a natural compound called cineole, which can increase blood flow in areas where it is applied topically (as an oil).

CHILES. Eating chiles generates physiological responses in our bodies (e.g., sweating, increased heart rate and circulation) that are similar to those experienced when having sex. The capsaicin in chiles is responsible for the effects. Do not touch your skin anywhere (including the genitals) after touching chiles because these foods are irritants to the skin.

GARLIC. Long ago, Tibetan monks were not allowed to enter the monastery if they had been eating garlic because of its reputation for stirring up passions. Garlic increases circulation and helps prevent hardening of the arteries, which can be a frequent cause of impotence in men. The downside of garlic is bad breath, so enjoy your garlic-laden foods long before you hit the bedroom.

GINGER. People have deemed ginger an aphrodisiac for centuries because of its scent and because it stimulates the circulatory system.

HONEY. In medioval times, people drank mead, a fermented drink made from honey, to boost sexual desire. Honey is loaded with B vitamins (needed for testosterone production) as well as boron (which helps the body metabolize and use estrogen). Some studies have suggested that it may also enhance blood levels of testosterone.

LICORICE. In ancient China, people used licorice to enhance love and

continued

lust. The smell appears to be particularly stimulating. In a study of how different smells stimulate sexual desire, researchers found that the smell of black licorice increased blood flow to the penis by 13 percent. When combined with the smell of doughnuts, that percentage jumped to 32.

PINE NUTS. People have been using pine nuts to stimulate libido since medieval times. Like oysters, they are high in zinc. Pine nuts have been included in love potions for centuries. The medical scholar Galen recommended eating one hundred pine nuts before going to bed.

STARTERS AND OTHER DELIGHTS

Fig Banana Smoothie

1 cup chopped dried figs
1 cup nonfat plain yogurt
1 tablespoon honey
1 cup sliced banana
3 cups crushed ice
Mint leaves or berries, to garnish

Place all the ingredients except the garnish in a blender and blend until smooth, 2 to 3 minutes. Strain and pour into chilled tall glasses, garnish, and serve immediately.

Makes 4 servings

Source: Centers for Disease Control

Nectarine and Basil Bagel

2 bagels, split
4 tablespoons fat-free cream cheese
12 large basil leaves
2 nectarines, thinly sliced
¼ teaspoon cracked black pepper

Toast the bagels and spread with the cream cheese. Top with the basil leaves and nectarine slices. Sprinkle with the pepper and serve.

Makes 2 servings

Source: Centers for Disease Control

Golden Apple Oatmeal

1 Golden Delicious apple, diced
⅓ cup apple juice
⅓ cup water
Dash of ground nutmeg
Dash of ground cinnamon
⅓ cup quick-cooking rolled oats

In a small saucepan, combine the apple, apple juice, water, nutmeg, and cinnamon. Place over medium heat and bring to a boil. Stir in the rolled oats and cook for 1 minute. Cover and let stand about 5 minutes before serving.

Makes 1 serving

Source: Centers for Disease Control

Green Chile Dip

One 16-ounce container lowfat cottage cheese
2 teaspoons fresh lemon juice
2 cups nonfat plain yogurt
1 cup frozen green chiles, defrosted and drained,
*   liquid reserved*
1 tablespoon garlic powder
½ teaspoon ground cumin
1 tablespoon dried oregano
1 teaspoon black pepper
1 teaspoon chili powder
Carrot and jicama slices, to serve

In a blender or food processor, combine the cottage cheese
and lemon juice and blend until smooth. Add the yogurt and
blend until smooth. In large bowl, combine the cottage cheese
mixture, the chiles, garlic powder, cumin, oregano, and black pepper. Gently stir until mixed well. If too stiff, stir in some of the
green chile juice. Cover and refrigerate for at least 2 hours before serving. Just before serving, sprinkle the chili powder on
top. Serve with carrot and jicama slices.

Makes 5 cups

Source: U.S. Department of Health and Human Services, Indian Health,
Division of Diabetes Treatment and Prevention

Bruschetta with Plums and Fresh Basil

One 24-inch sourdough baguette
4 ounces whipped fat-free cream cheese

6 cups sliced fresh plums
1 cup fresh basil leaves, to garnish

Preheat the oven to 350°F. Slice the baguette into 1-inch-thick pieces. Place on a baking sheet and toast in the oven until golden brown, about 3 to 5 minutes. Spread each slice of bread with cream cheese and place several plum slices on each piece of bruschetta. Garnish with basil leaves.

Makes 6 servings

Source: Centers for Disease Control

SMART SIDE DISHES

Papaya Black Beans and Rice

2 teaspoons olive oil
½ cup fresh orange juice
2 tablespoons chopped fresh cilantro
1 cup finely chopped red bell pepper
1 cup finely chopped green bell pepper
1 medium papaya, peeled, seeded, and diced
1 cup chopped red onion
¼ cup fresh lemon juice
½ teaspoon cayenne pepper
2 cloves garlic, minced
Two 15-ounce cans black beans, rinsed and drained
6 cups hot cooked brown rice

Heat the oil in a large skillet over medium heat. Add all the ingredients except the beans and rice. Cook for 5 minutes, stirring occasionally, until the bell peppers are crisp-tender. Stir in the beans and cook for about 5 minutes, or until heated through.

Makes 6 servings

Source: Centers for Disease Control

Green Chile Cornbread

1 cup all-purpose flour
1 cup cornmeal
4 teaspoons baking powder
¼ cup sugar
1 teaspoon salt
¼ cup vegetable oil
2 large eggs
1 cup milk
½ cup canned green chiles
½ cup grated cheddar cheese

Preheat the oven to 400°F. Grease a 12×12-inch baking dish.

In a large bowl, combine the flour, cornmeal, baking powder, sugar, and salt. In a separate bowl, whisk together the oil, eggs, and milk. Stir the wet ingredients into the dry and add the chiles and cheese. Mix thoroughly and pour into the baking dish. Bake for 20 minutes, or until golden brown. Cool prior to serving.

Makes 24 slices

Source: U.S. Department of Health and Human Services, Indian Health, Division of Diabetes Treatment and Prevention

Cranberry Salad

One 4-serving package sugar-free raspberry gelatin
One 4-serving package vanilla cook-and-serve pudding
1 cup water
2 cups fresh cranberries
¾ cup nonfat plain yogurt
⅓ cup nonfat dry milk powder
Sugar substitute to equal 2 tablespoons sugar
1 teaspoon vanilla extract
½ cup whipped topping
2 cups (from about 2 medium) diced bananas

In a medium saucepan, combine the dry gelatin and pudding mix. Stir in the water and cranberries. Place over medium heat and cook, stirring constantly, until the mixture comes to a boil and the cranberries soften. Remove from the heat, place the pan on a wire rack, and cool for 30 minutes. In a large bowl, combine the yogurt and dry milk powder. Stir in the sugar substitute and vanilla. Fold in the whipped topping. Add the cooled cranberry mixture and diced bananas and mix gently to combine. Evenly spoon the mixture into 6 serving dishes, cover with plastic, and refrigerate for at least 30 minutes before serving.

Makes 6 servings

Source: U.S. Department of Health and Human Services, Indian Health,
Division of Diabetes Treatment and Prevention

Artichoke Heart and Asparagus Salad with Strawberry Dressing

SALAD

6 lettuce leaves
6 small artichokes, cooked
1 pound fresh asparagus, cooked and chilled
⅓ cup shredded carrot

DRESSING

½ cup buttermilk
2 teaspoons honey
1 cup sliced fresh strawberries
¼ teaspoon ground allspice

To make the salad, arrange the lettuce leaves on 6 salad plates. Halve the artichokes lengthwise; remove the center petals and fuzzy centers and discard. Remove the outer leaves of the artichokes and reserve to use as a garnish. Trim out the hearts and slice. Arrange the artichoke slices on lettuce leaves, along with the asparagus and shredded carrot. Garnish with a few artichoke leaves.

For the dressing, in a blender or food processor, combine all the dressing ingredients and blend until smooth. Spoon the dressing over the salads and serve. The salad can be prepared up to 4 hours before serving time; cover the arranged salad plates and keep in the refrigerator until ready to serve. Spoon on the dressing just before serving.

Makes 6 servings

Source: Centers for Disease Control

Asian Salad

1 bay spring salad lettuce mix
½ cup lowfat vinaigrette of your choice
1 papaya, peeled, pitted, and thinly sliced
1 Asian pear, peeled, cored, and julienned
1 guava, peeled and thinly sliced

Place the greens in a large bowl and toss with dressing. Mound on a platter, arrange the fruit slices on top, and serve.

Makes 4 servings

Source: Centers for Disease Control

Chayote and Poblano Stew

½ cup pineapple juice
1 tablespoon olive oil
1 large chayote squash, peeled, halved lengthwise,
   and pitted
1 large cucumber, halved lengthwise and thinly sliced
4 poblano chiles, roasted, peeled, and thinly sliced
2 cups diced fresh pineapple
1 tablespoon Dijon-style mustard

In a small saucepan, simmer the pineapple juice over medium-low heat until it is reduced to 2 tablespoons. Transfer to a small bowl and let cool to room temperature.

Heat the oil in a medium skillet over medium heat. Add the chayote and sauté until crisp-tender, 1 to 2 minutes. In a large bowl, combine the chayotes, cucumber, chiles, and pineapple.

Whisk the pineapple juice with the mustard and pour over vegetables. Mix well. Serve immediately.

Makes 8 servings

Source: Centers for Disease Control

Lima Bean Salad with Garlic-Herb Dressing

DRESSING

3 tablespoons olive oil

3 tablespoons red wine vinegar

½ tablespoon honey

⅛ teaspoon ground nutmeg

½ teaspoon salt

2 tablespoons chopped green onion

1 tablespoon minced fresh tarragon or 1 teaspoon dried tarragon

3 cloves garlic, minced or pressed

SALAD

5 cups cooked baby lima beans (from 1¾ cups dry)

⅓ cup finely chopped fresh parsley

To make the dressing, in a medium bowl, whisk together all the dressing ingredients.

To make the salad, in a large bowl, combine the lima beans and parsley. Toss with the dressing. Let stand at room temperature for 1 hour before serving or cover and refrigerate for up to 6 hours, bringing to room temperature before serving.

Makes 4 servings

Source: Centers for Disease Control

Marinated Edamame Salad

DRESSING

2 tablespoons olive oil

2 tablespoons water

¼ cup fresh lemon juice

¼ cup white wine vinegar

1 tablespoon honey

2 tablespoons Dijon-style mustard

2 cloves garlic, minced

¼ teaspoon dried basil

¼ teaspoon dried marjoram

¼ teaspoon dried rosemary

¼ teaspoon dried thyme

¼ teaspoon black pepper

¼ teaspoon grated lemon zest

SALAD

2 cups green beans, trimmed and cut into bite-size pieces,
    lightly cooked

¼ cup diced green onion

½ cup diced celery

2 tablespoons minced fresh parsley

2 cups cooked and shelled edamame

½ cup chopped red bell pepper

½ cup chopped cucumber

1 cup chopped carrots

⅓ cup dried cranberries

2 cups chopped romaine lettuce

To make the dressing, in a medium bowl, whisk together the oil, water, lemon juice, vinegar, honey, mustard, garlic, basil, marjoram, rosemary, thyme, black pepper, and lemon zest. Set aside.

To make the salad, in a salad bowl, toss together all of the salad ingredients except the lettuce. Whisk the dressing again, pour over the salad, and toss. Cover and refrigerate for at least 1 hour before serving. When ready to serve, arrange the lettuce on salad plates and top with the salad mixture.

Makes 8 servings

Source: Centers for Disease Control

Vegetable Stew

3 cups water

1 cube low-sodium vegetable bouillon

2 cups white potatoes cut into 2-inch strips

2 cups sliced carrots

4 cups summer squash cut in 1-inch squares

1 cup summer squash cut in 4 chunks

One 15-ounce can corn kernels, rinsed and drained, or 1½ cups fresh corn kernels

1 teaspoon dried thyme

2 cloves garlic, minced

1 scallion, chopped

½ small hot chile, chopped

1 cup coarsely chopped onion

1 cup diced tomatoes

Place the water and bouillon cube in a large pot. Place over high heat and bring to a boil, stirring to dissolve the bouillon. Add the potatoes and carrots, bring to a simmer, reduce the heat to medium, and simmer for 5 minutes. Add the remaining ingredients except the tomatoes and cooking for an additional 15 minutes. Remove 4 chunks of the squash and purée in a blender. Return the puréed squash to the pot and cook for 10 minutes. Add the tomatoes and cook for another 5 minutes, or until all the vegetables have softened. Remove from the heat and let sit for 10 minutes for the stew to thicken, then serve.

Makes 8 servings

Source: National Institutes of Health, National Heart,
Lung, and Blood Institute

BRAIN POWER ENTRÉES

Scalloped Oysters and Fennel

1 fennel bulb, about 12 ounces
3½ tablespoons unsalted butter
1 pint oysters with their liquor
2 tablespoons fresh lemon juice
1½ cups dried breadcrumbs
Salt and black pepper

Preheat the oven to 425°F and butter a shallow, 8-inch ovenproof dish.

Trim the root and leaves from the fennel bulb and reserve some of the feathery leaves for garnish. Quarter the bulb and cut it across into thin slices; cut the root into julienne. Melt 2 tablespoons of the butter in a sauté pan over medium-low heat, add the fennel, and sauté, stirring, for about 5 minutes, or until softened. Drain the oysters into a small bowl, saving the liquor and adding the lemon juice to it. When the fennel has cooled somewhat, mix it with the oysters.

Scatter a third of the breadcrumbs in the bottom of the baking dish. Cover with half the oyster-fennel mixture, then scatter another third of breadcrumbs over it. Layer the remaining oyster-fennel mixture, then spread the remaining breadcrumbs on top. Spoon over the reserved oyster liquor, dot with the remaining butter, and add salt and pepper to taste. Place in the oven and bake for 25 minutes, or until golden brown and bubbling. Garnish with the reserved fennel leaves and serve immediately.

Makes 4 servings

Recipe courtesy of the Pacific Coast Shellfish
Growers Association

Main Dish Vegetarian Salad

½ head red cabbage, cored and thickly sliced
½ head romaine lettuce, torn into pieces
3 medium carrots, grated or sliced
1 cucumber, sliced
1 green bell pepper, chopped
2 stalks broccoli, cut into florets
3 medium tomatoes, cut into wedges
Two 16-ounce cans kidney beans or chickpeas
6 ounces grated reduced-fat cheddar cheese
¼ cup fat-free Italian or French salad dressing

In a large bowl, combine all the salad ingredients. Just before serving, toss with the salad dressing and serve.

Makes 8 servings

Source: Food Stamp Nutrition Connection

Salmon Loaf

One 15½-ounce can salmon
2 cups soft breadcrumbs
1 large onion, chopped
1 tablespoon melted margarine
¼ cup diced celery
1 cup lowfat milk
1 tablespoon fresh lemon juice
1 teaspoon dried parsley
2 large eggs

Preheat the oven to 325°F. Lightly oil a 9×5-inch loaf pan.

Drain the salmon and remove the skin if you like. Place in a large bowl and mash the bones with the meat. Add the other ingredients with enough milk so that the mixture is moist but not runny. Bake for 45 minutes, or until loaf is brown on top. Cut into slices and serve.

Makes 4 servings

Source: Food Stamp Nutrition Connection

Scrumptious Meatloaf

1 pound extra-lean ground beef
½ cup tomato paste

¼ cup finely chopped onion

¼ cup finely chopped green bell peppers

¼ cup finely chopped red bell peppers

1 cup peeled chopped tomatoes

½ teaspoon low-sodium prepared mustard

¼ teaspoon black pepper

½ teaspoon chopped chile

2 cloves garlic, minced

2 scallions, finely chopped

½ teaspoon ground ginger

⅛ teaspoon ground nutmeg

1 teaspoon grated orange zest

½ teaspoon crushed thyme

¼ cup fine breadcrumbs

Preheat the oven to 350°F.

In a large bowl, mix all the ingredients together. Place in a loaf pan (preferably a pan with a drip rack), cover with foil, and bake for 50 minutes. Uncover the pan and continue baking for about 12 minutes, or until meat is done throughout. Remove from the oven, slice, and serve.

Makes 6 servings

Source: National Heart, Lung, and Blood Institute

ENERGIZING DESSERTS

Fresh Orange Compote with Granola

2 navel oranges, peeled and separated into segments

1 apple or pear, peeled, cored, and diced

1 banana, thinly sliced
½ cup halved seedless red or green grapes
2 tablespoons fresh orange juice
½ cup lowfat granola

In a medium bowl, toss together orange segments, apple, banana, grapes, and orange juice. Sprinkle the granola over the mixture and toss lightly. Serve immediately.

Makes 6 servings

Source: Centers for Disease Control

Papaya Boats

2 ripe papayas
1 small ripe banana, sliced
1 cup canned mandarin orange segments, drained
1 kiwi, peeled and sliced
½ cup fresh blueberries
½ cup fresh strawberry slices
¾ cup nonfat vanilla yogurt
2 teaspoons chopped fresh mint, plus mint sprigs, to garnish
    (optional)

Cut the papayas in half lengthwise and scoop out the seeds. Place the banana, oranges, kiwi, blueberries, and strawberries in each papaya half. In a small bowl, combine the yogurt and mint; mix well and spoon over the fruit before serving. Garnish with mint sprigs, if using.

Makes 4 servings

Source: Centers for Disease Control

Watermelon-Blueberry Banana Split

2 large bananas
8 watermelon scoops (watermelon balls formed with an ice
    cream scoop)
2 cups fresh blueberries
½ cup lowfat vanilla yogurt
¼ cup lowfat granola

Peel the bananas and cut in half crosswise, then cut each piece in half lengthwise. For each serving, lay 2 banana pieces against the sides of a shallow dish. Place a watermelon scoop at each end of the dish. Fill the center space with blueberries. Stir the yogurt until smooth and spoon over the watermelon scoops. Sprinkle with the granola and serve.

Makes 4 servings

Source: Centers for Disease Control

Banana and Yogurt Crêpes

¾ cup lowfat milk
¾ cup all-purpose flour
1 large egg
1 large egg white
2 tablespoons honey or maple syrup
One 8-ounce container lowfat banana or vanilla yogurt
½ teaspoon vanilla extract
1 banana, diced
Fresh mint sprigs, to garnish (optional)
Powdered sugar, to garnish (optional)

In a medium bowl, whisk together the milk, flour, egg, egg white, and 1 tablespoon of the honey. Set aside the batter to rest for 5 minutes at room temperature. Heat a 10-inch non-stick skillet over medium heat. Pour ¼ cup of the batter into skillet; quickly tilt and swirl the batter to coat the bottom of the skillet. When the crêpe is lightly browned at edges, use a thin spatula to loosen and turn over. Cook about 20 seconds on the other side, until lightly browned, then slide onto a plate to cool. Continue making crêpes with the remaining batter. To prevent sticking, place a piece of wax paper between each crêpe.

In a blender or food processor, combine the yogurt, vanilla, and remaining 1 tablespoon honey and blend until smooth. Add the diced banana. Spread each crêpe with about 2½ tablespoons of the yogurt mixture and roll the crêpes into cylinders. Place 2 crêpes on each serving plate and garnish with mint sprigs and powdered sugar, if using.

Makes 4 servings

Recipe courtesy of Dairy Management Inc.

Cocoa-Berry Yogurt Tarts

1½ cups lowfat vanilla yogurt
1½ cups reduced-fat ricotta cheese
2 tablespoons sugar
2 tablespoons unsweetened cocoa powder
6 small graham cracker tart shells
¾ cup sliced strawberries (or substitute raspberries or blueberries)

In a medium bowl, whisk together the yogurt, ricotta, sugar, and cocoa powder until creamy. Spoon one sixth of the mixture into each tart shell and top with the sliced strawberries. Refrigerate for 4 hours.

Makes 6 servings

Recipe courtesy of Dairy Management Inc.

RESOURCES

Thank you to the following trade associations and companies who generously contributed recipes to this book. We've included Web site information on each one so that you can find more great recipes, food preparation tips, and nutritional information to help you live a healthier lifestyle.

American Egg Board
www.aeb.org

The American Egg Board (AEB) is the U.S. egg producer's link to the consumer in communicating the nutritional value of the incredible egg. As the egg industry's promotional arm, AEB's challenges are to convince the American public that the egg is still one of nature's most nearly perfect foods and to improve the demand for eggs and egg products throughout the United States.

American Lamb Board
www.americanlambboard.org

The American Lamb Board (ALB) was created by the U.S. Secretary of Agriculture. The ALB works to strengthen the domestic lamb industry's position in the marketplace through advertising, public relations, culinary education, and retail promotions. The thirteen-member volunteer board represents all sectors of the lamb industry in the United States.

Bumble Bee
www.bumblebee.com

Bumble Bee Foods was founded by a handful of dedicated canners back in 1899. As an international company, Bumble Bee employs over a thousand men and women and sells canned tuna, salmon, and other seafood throughout the world under the Bumble Bee label and in Canada under the Clover Leaf brand name. The company has canning facilities in Mayagüez, Puerto Rico, and Santa Fe Springs, California.

California Dried Plum Board
www.californiadriedplums.org

The California Dried Plum Board represents a thousand dried plum growers and twenty-two dried plum packers under the authority of the U.S. Secretary of Food and Agriculture to direct and manage activities in four areas: advertising, public relations, and sales promotion; market research; production, processing, and nutrition research; and education.

California Fresh Figs Growers Association
www.calfreshfigs.com

The California Fresh Figs Growers Association represents the growers and shippers of various species of figs in California.

California Salmon Council
www.calkingsalmon.org

The California Salmon Council was formed in 1989 to represent the marketing interests of the state's commercial salmon fishermen. The Council's goal is to create consumer awareness and marketplace demand for California King Salmon.

Calorie Control Council
www.caloriecontrol.org

The Calorie Control Council is an excellent source of information on cutting calories and fat in your diet, achieving and maintaining a healthy weight, and using your favorite low-calorie, reduced-fat foods and beverages to stay fit and healthy.

Cape Cod Cranberry Growers' Association
www.cranberries.org

Established in 1888 to standardize the measure with which cranberries are sold, the Cape Cod Cranberry Growers' Association (CCCGA) is one of the country's oldest farmers' organizations. Today the CCCGA represents approximately 330 growers throughout Massachusetts to help promote the cranberry industry.

Chilean Fresh Fruit Association
www.cffa.org

This organization aims to promote Chile as a leading fresh fruit exporter, using information about the quality and health of their products to do so. It also develops networks for Chile in the world market.

Chocolate Council (of the National Confectioners Association)
www.chocolateusa.org

The Council (formerly the Chocolate Manufacturers Association) has served as the premier trade group for manufacturers and distributors of cocoa and chocolate products in the United States since 1923. The association was founded to fund and administer research, promote chocolate to the general public, and serve as an advocate of the industry before Congress and government agencies.

Concord Grape Association

www.concordgrape.org

The Concord Grape Association represents processors of Concords and manufacturers of products derived from Concords. The organization operates as the Concord Grape Section under the umbrella of the Juice Products Association (JPA), which represents the juice and juice products industry in the United States and overseas. Concord Grape Section members handle more than the majority of the Concord grapes processed annually in the United States. The Concord Grape Association meets routinely to share information on a wide range of issues, including authenticity, projected crop size, crop quality, and research regarding the health benefits of grapes and grape products.

Dairy Management Inc.

www.3aday.org

Dairy Management Inc. is the nonprofit domestic and international planning and management organization responsible for increasing demand for U.S.-produced dairy products on behalf of America's dairy farmers. DMI manages the American Dairy Association, National Dairy Council, and U.S. Dairy Export Council. DMI also promotes the 3-A-Day of Dairy to consumers. Research shows that on average, Americans are eating only half the daily recommended servings of dairy. 3-A-Day of Dairy was thus created as a simple reminder for families to get three daily servings of milk, cheese, or yogurt for stronger bones and better bodies. Dairy provides nine essential nutrients, including calcium; potassium; phosphorus; protein; vitamins A, D, and B_{12}; riboflavin; and niacin (niacin equivalents).

Florida Department of Citrus Headquarters

www.Floridajuice.com

This state organization is responsible for the correct labeling of citrus fruit from Florida and guarantees appropriate quality of the products. It is primarily involved in increasing the quality and quantity of citrus fruits. It also provides education about the many uses of the fruit across broad bands of applications.

Georgia Fruit and Vegetable Growers Association
www.gfvga.org

The Georgia Fruit and Vegetable Growers Association's (GFVGA) mission is to provide a united voice to represent an industry that is valued in excess of $700 million dollars. Most Georgia fruits and vegetables are grown for the fresh market to be sold and consumed in other states. The GFVGA provides programs and services to its membership designed to increase production efficiencies, provide educational opportunities, promote new markets, monitor legislation, encourage applied research, and improve communications among GFVGA members and industry suppliers.

Hawaii Papaya Industry Association
www.hawaiipapaya.com

The Hawaii Papaya Industry Association promotes nutritious, quality Hawaii-grown papayas to consumers worldwide. The association exists to promote the improvement of business conditions in the state of Hawaii for the papaya industry, including the conditions relating to cultivation, distribution, sales, and use of papayas.

Idaho Barley Commission
www.idahobarley.org

The Idaho Barley Commission (IBC) is a self-governing agency of the state of Idaho that serves to enhance the profitability of Idaho barley growers through research, market development, promotion, information, and education. This is accomplished by identifying and fully utilizing available resources and organizations to promote and further develop the barley industry in the state of Idaho.

Manitoba Canola Growers Association

www.mcgacanola.org

The Manitoba Canola Growers Association (MCGA) is an organization committed to maximizing net income from canola. It helps growers with production, marketing, market development for canola products, and awareness of the benefits of canola.

Michigan Blueberry Growers Association

www.blueberries.com

The Michigan Blueberry Growers Association is a producer-owned blueberry marketing cooperative that was formed in 1936 as Michigan Blueberry Growers by the original blueberry growers in the state. Today, with a production base of over 550 growers and total annual sales in excess of $63 million, the association is the single largest marketer of fresh and processed cultivated blueberries in the world.

Midwest Dairy Association

www.midwestdairy.com

Midwest Dairy Association (MDA) is a nonprofit organization that is financed and directed by the dairy producers in nine states— Arkansas, Illinois, Iowa, Kansas, Minnesota, Missouri, North Dakota, South Dakota, and eastern Oklahoma. It implements programs that help increase sales and demand for dairy products and dairy ingredients to help improve the economic well-being of Midwest dairy producers. The Midwest Dairy Council (MDC), the nutrition marketing arm of the Midwest Dairy Association, works with teachers, school nutrition departments, and community leaders to develop sound and effective dairy nutrition education programs.

Minnesota Pork Board

www.mnpork.com

This organization is dedicated to training in productive pork products and healthy animal care. Education is a major force within the organization for healthy approaches to the development of pigs. Interest in food preparation using pork is also a major mission.

National Coffee Association of U.S.A., Inc.

www.ncausa.org

The National Coffee Association of U.S.A. was founded in 1911, one of the earliest trade associations formed in the United States and the first trade association for the U.S. coffee industry. Since that time, the NCA has helped American coffee companies through some of the most volatile periods in the nation's history, including two world wars, a depression, a cold war, and numerous frosts, strikes, and cartels, not to mention a wide range of consumer trends in the U.S. coffee market. Its members are found throughout the United States and overseas. They include retailers in California, importers in Tennessee, roasters in Ohio, suppliers in Illinois, and wholesalers in New York, as well as market exchanges, associations, and exporters operating on every continent.

National Turkey Federation

www.eatturkey.com

The National Turkey Federation is the national advocate for all segments of the turkey industry, providing services and conducting activities that increase demand for its members' products by protecting and enhancing their ability to profitably provide wholesome, high-quality, nutritious products.

National Watermelon Promotion Board

www.watermelon.org

The National Watermelon Promotion Board (NWPB) operates with a single objective: to increase consumer demand for watermelon through promotion, research, and educational programs. The Orlando-based nonprofit organization was formed in 1989 by watermelon growers and shippers. Since then, the NWPB has developed marketing programs to boost watermelon sales in supermarkets throughout the United States and Canada. Through high profile publicity on television, radio, newspapers, and magazines, the board has showcased watermelon as a healthy, refreshing, versatile fruit. Thanks in part to board efforts, watermelon is not only for picnics anymore, but has won a regular place on consumers' shopping lists enjoyed year-round in slices or added to a wide variety of desserts, drinks, and other recipes.

Nevada Waterfowl Association

www.nevadawaterfowl.org

The Nevada Waterfowl Association's mission is to protect, restore, and enhance Nevada's wetlands and the wildlife dependent upon them, especially waterfowl and shorebirds. The Nevada Waterfowl Association works closely with organizations such as the U.S. Fish & Wildlife Service, Nevada Division of Wildlife, Lahontan Wetlands Coalition, The Nature Conservancy, Ducks Unlimited, and other conservation organizations that share their goal of preserving Nevada's unique desert wetlands for future generations to enjoy.

North American Bramble Growers Association

www.raspberryblackberry.com

The North American Bramble Growers Association (NABGA) is a membership association of blackberry and raspberry growers and agricultural professionals. Its Web site has information for consumers and media, growers and researchers, kids, and more.

North American Millers' Association

www.namamillers.org

The North American Millers' Association (NAMA) is the trade association of the wheat, corn, oat, and rye milling industry. It is comprised of milling member companies operating mills in the United States and Canada and associate member companies representing the industries providing products and services to the mills. The aggregate production capacity of NAMA milling members is more than 160 million pounds of product daily, which is about 95 percent of the total U.S. capacity.

Northarvest Bean Growers Association

www.northarvestbean.org

The Northarvest Bean Growers Association represents the growers of America's heartland who grow top-quality beans. The association supplies market news and bean reports, as well as research and production information. It also publishes a magazine, the *Northarvest Bean Grower*, in which you can learn more about the industry.

North Carolina Sweet Potato Commission

www.ncsweetpotatoes.com

The North Carolina Sweet Potato Commission is a nonprofit corporation chartered on June 30, 1961, by six sweet potato farmers. For more than forty years, North Carolina farmers have sought to increase sweet potato consumption by collectively funding promotional programs, providing timely and relevant information to themselves as well as consumers, funding research and development projects, and encouraging the use of good seed stock and horticultural practices among producers.

Northern Canola Growers Association

www.northerncanola.com

The mission of the Northern Canola Growers Association is to promote and encourage the establishment and maintenance of conditions favorable to the production, marketing, processing, research, and use of canola; to promote efficient production through farmer education, public and private research, labeling, and registration of crop protection products; to promote uniform seed and product standards; and to work to develop and implement agriculture policies that will enhance development of the industry.

Northern Plains Potato Growers Association

www.rrvpotatoes.org

This organization promotes the profitability and unity of the potato growers of the adjacent states and North Dakota. The quality of the potato is a major goal, with research and educational programs. The increase in ways of food preparation is always nurtured. The production of excellence in developing new techniques and genetic brands of potatoes is a major interest.

Oregon Raspberry and Blackberry Commission

www.oregon-berries.com

The Oregon Raspberry and Blackberry Commission (ORBC) was established in 1981. At that time the commission was called the Oregon Caneberry Commission. After years of struggling with public confusion over the term "caneberry," the commission changed its name in 1992. Caneberries are berries that grow on a cane, such as raspberries, blackberries, marionberries, and boysenberries. The commission consists of nine members: six growers, two processors, and one public member. Their primary focus is promotion of caneberries. Strong secondary directions are research and education. The ORBC has more than 550 growers in Oregon.

Pacific Coast Shellfish Growers Association

www.pcsga.org

Founded in 1930, the Pacific Coast Shellfish Growers Association (PCSGA) represents growers in Alaska, Washington, Oregon, California, and Hawaii. The members of PCSGA grow a wide variety of healthy, sustainable shellfish, including oysters, clams, mussels, scallops, and geoduck.

Pioneer Valley Growers Association

www.pvga.net

The Pioneer Valley Growers Association is a cooperative of farmers located in the Pioneer Valley of Western Massachusetts. The PVGA distributes fruit and produce grown by local farmers to supermarket chains within Massachusetts and throughout New England. The mission of the PVGA is to provide consumers with the freshest, highest-quality locally grown produce. The farmland in the Pioneer Valley has some of the richest soil in the world. This, combined with state-of-the-art cooling technology, allows its farmers to produce some of the finest looking and best tasting vegetables around.

R.C. Bigelow
www.bigelowtea.com

R.C. Bigelow is a family-owned company that makes quality tea. Its goal is to "make sure you get the best tasting cup of tea possible." Because flavor is so important, every tea bag is overwrapped and sealed in a stay-fresh foil packet so that all the goodness stays in until you get ready to have a cup of tea.

Restaurant Association of Maryland
www.marylandrestaurants.com

The Restaurant Association of Maryland helps elect and re-elect pro-business candidates to the Maryland General Assembly. Effective lobbying efforts protect the industry from taxes or regulations that would negatively impact the industry. Legislative victories have resulted in saving the average Maryland restaurant owner more than $100,000 annually.

Revival Soy
www.soyfoods.com

Revival Soy is a line of soy products made by Physicians Laboratories to serve customers with good nutrition, education, and medical research. Physicians Laboratories was founded by Dr. Aaron Tabor, M.D., in an effort to help his mother, Suzanne, with her menopausal transition. He accomplished this goal by creating patented Revival

Soy. Revival Soy has been shipping since 1998 with more that 1,000,000 orders shipped to over 300,000 unique customers. The company's 56,000-square-foot facility is located in Kernersville, North Carolina.

Sunsweet Growers Inc.
www.sunsweet.com

Sunsweet Growers is the world's largest handler of dried tree fruits, including cranberries, apricots, and prunes. A grower-owned marketing cooperative representing more than a third of the prune market worldwide, Sunsweet processes more than 50,000 tons of prunes a year. Founded in 1917 as the California Prune and Apricot Growers Association, the cooperative served as a marketing agent to offer the crops of its members—under the brand name Sunsweet—to consumers at better prices than were offered by individual growers. Today Sunsweet processes and markets the dried fruit production of more than four hundred grower-members with orchard holdings primarily in California's Sacramento and San Joaquin valleys. After nearly nine decades, Sunsweet boasts an enviable brand recognition of 85 percent in American households, placing it in the very top rank of long-standing successful American products.

Turbana Corporation
www.turbana.com

Turbana Corporation is a banana producer that originated from the independent growers of Colombia's Urabá region. In the 1960s, those growers came together to form the Unibán cooperative, which eventually became Turbana's corporate parent. Turbana started as a small importer in 1970; now it is one of the top labels in North America. Today Unibán grows, packs, ships, and markets more than 30 percent of the bananas grown in Colombia under the Turbana label. Turbana is the fourth largest importer of bananas and the first importer of plantains in North America.

USA Dry Pea and Lentil Council

www.pea-lentil.com

The USA Dry Pea and Lentil Council is a nonprofit organization founded in 1965 for the purpose of promoting and protecting those engaged in growing, processing, warehousing, and merchandising peas, lentils, and chickpeas. The Council represents more than five thousand growers, processors, exporters, and associates of premium commodities.

Walnut Marketing Board

www.walnuts.org

The Walnut Marketing Board was established in 1933 to represent the walnut growers and handlers of California. The board is funded by mandatory assessments of the handlers. The WMB is governed by a Federal Walnut Marketing Order. The board promotes the use of walnuts in the United States through publicity and educational programs. The board also provides funding for walnut production and post-harvest research.

Wheat Foods Council

www.wheatfoods.org

The Wheat Foods Council is a national nonprofit organization formed in 1972 to help increase awareness of dietary grains as an essential component to a healthy diet. The Council continues to counteract media misinformation as well as further educate the public on the goodness of both enriched and whole grain foods.

Wholesome Sweeteners

www.wholesomesweeteners.com

Wholesome Sweeteners supplies Fair Trade Certified organic and natural sugars, syrups, and nectars to North American retail and industrial markets. Wholesome supplies only the finest organic and natural sugar products from ethically and environmentally responsible growers and manufacturers and provides consumers with the choice of flavorful, organic, and natural sugars that are produced with respect for the planet and people and utmost concern for food safety and the health and nutritional needs of consumers and their families.

Other Valuable Resources and Web Sites

For other great recipes, check out these government Web sites:

- A Healthier You: www.hhs.gov
- Bureau of Markets/Farmers' Markets: www.mass.gov/agr/markets/farmersmarkets/index.htm
- Centers for Disease Control: www.fruitsandveggiesmatter.gov/month/index.html
- Food Stamp Nutrition Connection: recipefinder.nal.usda.gov
- National Institutes of Health; National Heart, Lung, and Blood Institute: www.nhlbi.nih.gov and www.nhlbi.nih.gov/health/public/heart/other/ktb_recipebk
- United States Department of Agriculture—Recipes and Tips for Healthy, Thrifty Meals: www.nutrition.gov
- United States Department of Health and Human Services, Indian Health, Division of Diabetes Treatment and Prevention: www.ihs.gov and www.smallstep.gov

INDEX